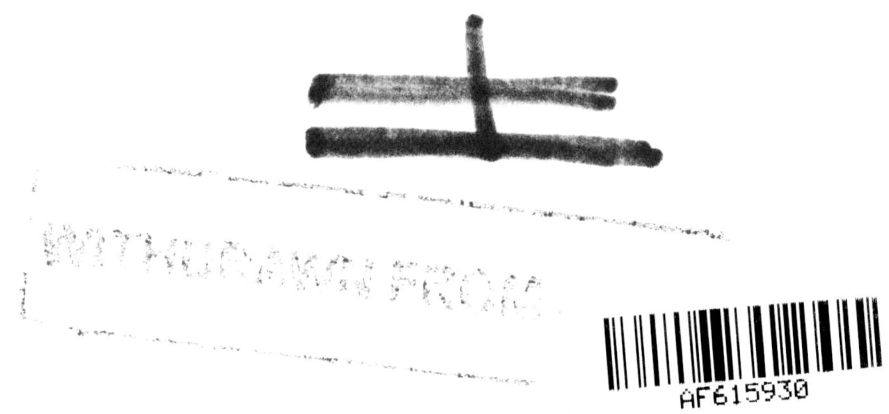

THE RECENT HISTORY OF PLATELETS IN THROMBOSIS AND OTHER DISORDERS

The transcript of a Witness Seminar held by the Wellcome Trust Centre for the History of Medicine at UCL, London, on 25 November 2003

Edited by L A Reynolds and E M Tansey

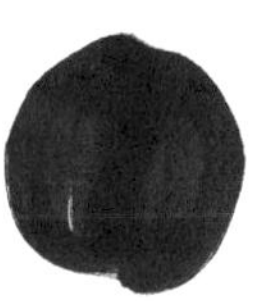

Volume 23 2005

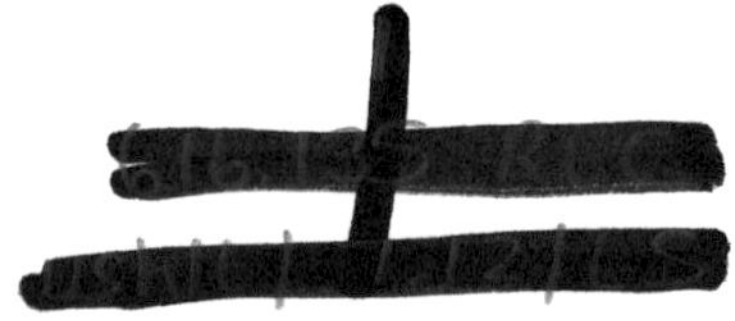

First published by the Wellcome Trust Centre
for the History of Medicine at UCL, 2005

The Wellcome Trust Centre for the History of Medicine
at University College London is funded by the Wellcome Trust,
which is a registered charity, no. 210183.

ISBN 0 85484 103 2

Histmed logo images courtesy of the Wellcome Library, London.

Design and production: Julie Wood at Shift Key Design 020 7241 3704

All volumes freely available following the links to publications at www.ucl.ac.uk/histmed

Technology Transfer in Britain: The case of monoclonal antibodies; Self and Non-Self: A history of autoimmunity; Endogenous Opiates; The Committee on Safety of Drugs • Making the Human Body Transparent: The impact of NMR and MRI; Research in General Practice; Drugs in Psychiatric Practice; The MRC Common Cold Unit • Early Heart Transplant Surgery in the UK • Haemophilia: Recent history of clinical management • Looking at the Unborn: Historical aspects of obstetric ultrasound • Post Penicillin Antibiotics: From acceptance to resistance? • Clinical Research in Britain, 1950–1980 • Intestinal Absorption • Origins of Neonatal Intensive Care in the UK • British Contributions to Medical Research and Education in Africa after the Second World War • Childhood Asthma and Beyond • Maternal Care • Population-based Research in South Wales: The MRC Pneumoconiosis Research Unit and the MRC Epidemiology Unit • Peptic Ulcer: Rise and fall • Leukaemia • The MRC Applied Psychology Unit • Genetic Testing • Foot and Mouth Disease: The 1967 outbreak and its aftermath • Environmental Toxicology: The legacy of *Silent Spring* • Cystic Fibrosis • Innovation in Pain Management • The Rhesus Factor and Disease Prevention

CONTENTS

ILLUSTRATIONS AND CREDITS

WITNESS SEMINARS: MEETINGS AND PUBLICATIONS[1]

In 1990 the Wellcome Trust created a History of Twentieth Century Medicine Group, as part of the Academic Unit of the Wellcome Institute for the History of Medicine, to bring together clinicians, scientists, historians and others interested in contemporary medical history. Among a number of other initiatives the format of Witness Seminars, used by the Institute of Contemporary British History to address issues of recent political history, was adopted, to promote interaction between these different groups, to emphasize the potential benefits of working jointly, and to encourage the creation and deposit of archival sources for present and future use. In June 1999 the Governors of the Wellcome Trust decided that it would be appropriate for the Academic Unit to enjoy a more formal academic affiliation and turned the Unit into the Wellcome Trust Centre for the History of Medicine at University College London from 1 October 2000. The Wellcome Trust continues to fund the Witness Seminar programme via its support for the Centre.

The Witness Seminar is a particularly specialized form of oral history, where several people associated with a particular set of circumstances or events are invited to come together to discuss, debate, and agree or disagree about their memories. To date, the History of Twentieth Century Medicine Group has held 40 such meetings, most of which have been published, as listed on pages xiii–xx.

Subjects are usually proposed by, or through, members of the Programme Committee of the Group, and once an appropriate topic has been agreed, suitable participants are identified and invited. This inevitably leads to further contacts, and more suggestions of people to invite. As the organization of the meeting progresses, a flexible outline plan for the meeting is devised, usually with assistance from the meeting's chairman, and some participants are invited to 'set the ball rolling' on particular themes, by speaking for a short period to initiate and stimulate further discussion.

Each meeting is fully recorded, the tapes are transcribed and the unedited transcript is immediately sent to every participant. Each is asked to check his or her own contributions and to provide brief biographical details. The editors

---

[1] The following text also appears in the 'Introduction' to recent volumes of *Wellcome Witnesses to Twentieth Century Medicine* published by the Wellcome Trust and the Wellcome Trust Centre for the History of Medicine at University College London.

turn the transcript into readable text, and participants' minor corrections and comments are incorporated into that text, while biographical and bibliographical details are added as footnotes, as are more substantial comments and additional material provided by participants. The final scripts are then sent to every contributor, accompanied by forms assigning copyright to the Wellcome Trust. Copies of all additional correspondence received during the editorial process are deposited with the records of each meeting in Archives and Manuscripts, Wellcome Library, London.

As with all our meetings, we hope that even if the precise details of some of the technical sections are not clear to the non-specialist, the sense and significance of the events will be understandable. Our aim is for the volumes that emerge from these meetings to inform those with a general interest in the history of modern medicine and medical science; to provide historians with new insights, fresh material for study, and further themes for research; and to emphasize to the participants that events of the recent past, of their own working lives, are of proper and necessary concern to historians.

ACKNOWLEDGEMENTS

'Platelets' was suggested as a suitable topic for a Witness Seminar by Professor Gustav Born and he provided many of the names of individuals to be invited, and assisted us in planning the meeting, and deciding the topics to be discussed. We are very grateful to him for his input. We are also indebted to Professor Tom Meade for writing such a useful Introduction to these published proceedings, and for his excellent chairing of the occasion. Our particular thanks go to Professors Gus Born and Tom Meade and Dr Jack Botting, who read through earlier drafts of the transcript, and offered us helpful comments and advice. We thank Professors Gus Born, John Hampton, Salvador Moncada, Peter Richardson and John Thompson, Dr Margaret Day and John Haynes for additional help with photographs; and Dr Mick Bakhle, Professor John Hampton, Dr Peter MacCallum, Dr Martyn Mahaut-Smith, Dr Robin Norris, Professor Peter Richardson and Dr Duncan Thomas for help with the Glossary.

As with all our meetings, we depend a great deal on our colleagues at the Wellcome Trust to ensure their smooth running: the Audiovisual Department, the Medical Photographic Library and Mrs Tracy Tillotson of the Wellcome Library; Ms Julie Wood, who has supervised the design and production of this volume; our indexer, Ms Liza Furnival, and our readers, Ms Lucy Moore and Mr Simon Reynolds. Mrs Jaqui Carter is our transcriber, and Mrs Wendy Kutner and Dr Daphne Christie assist us in running the meetings. Finally we thank the Wellcome Trust for supporting this programme.

Tilli Tansey

Lois Reynolds

Wellcome Trust Centre for the History of Medicine at UCL

HISTORY OF TWENTIETH CENTURY MEDICINE WITNESS SEMINARS, 1993–2005

1993 **Monoclonal antibodies**
Organizers: Dr E M Tansey and Dr Peter Catterall

1994 **The early history of renal transplantation**
Organizer: Dr Stephen Lock

Pneumoconiosis of coal workers
Organizer: Dr E M Tansey

1995 **Self and non-self: A history of autoimmunity**
Organizers: Sir Christopher Booth and Dr E M Tansey

Ashes to ashes: The history of smoking and health
Organizers: Dr Stephen Lock and Dr E M Tansey

Oral contraceptives
Organizers: Dr Lara Marks and Dr E M Tansey

Endogenous opiates
Organizer: Dr E M Tansey

1996 **Committee on Safety of Drugs**
Organizers: Dr Stephen Lock and Dr E M Tansey

Making the body more transparent: The impact of nuclear magnetic resonance and magnetic resonance imaging
Organizer: Sir Christopher Booth

1997 **Research in general practice**
Organizers: Dr Ian Tait and Dr E M Tansey

Drugs in psychiatric practice
Organizers: Dr David Healy and Dr E M Tansey

The MRC Common Cold Unit
Organizers: Dr David Tyrrell and Dr E M Tansey

The first heart transplant in the UK
Organizer: Professor Tom Treasure

1998	**Haemophilia: Recent history of clinical management** Organizers: Professor Christine Lee and Dr E M Tansey
	Obstetric ultrasound: Historical perspectives Organizers: Dr Malcolm Nicolson, Mr John Fleming and Dr E M Tansey
	Post penicillin antibiotics Organizers: Dr Robert Bud and Dr E M Tansey
	Clinical research in Britain, 1950–1980 Organizers: Dr David Gordon and Dr E M Tansey
1999	**Intestinal absorption** Organizers: Sir Christopher Booth and Dr E M Tansey
	The MRC Epidemiology Unit (South Wales) Organizers: Dr Andy Ness and Dr E M Tansey
	Neonatal intensive care Organizers: Professor Osmund Reynolds and Dr E M Tansey
	British contributions to medicine in Africa after the Second World War Organizers: Dr Mary Dobson, Dr Maureen Malowany, Dr Gordon Cook and Dr E M Tansey
2000	**Childhood asthma, and beyond** Organizers: Dr Chris O'Callaghan and Dr Daphne Christie
	Peptic ulcer: Rise and fall Organizers: Sir Christopher Booth, Professor Roy Pounder and Dr E M Tansey
	Maternal care Organizers: Dr Irvine Loudon and Dr Daphne Christie
2001	**Leukaemia** Organizers: Professor Sir David Weatherall, Professor John Goldman, Sir Christopher Booth and Dr Daphne Christie
	The MRC Applied Psychology Unit Organizers: Dr Geoff Bunn and Dr Daphne Christie
	Genetic testing Organizers: Professor Doris Zallen and Dr Daphne Christie

Foot and mouth disease: the 1967 outbreak and its aftermath
Organizers: Dr Abigail Woods, Dr Daphne Christie and Dr David Aickin

2002 **Environmental toxicology: The legacy of *Silent Spring***
Organizers: Dr Robert Flanagan and Dr Daphne Christie

Cystic fibrosis
Organizers: Dr James Littlewood and Dr Daphne Christie

Innovation in pain management
Organizers: Professor David Clark and Dr Daphne Christie

2003 **Thrombolysis**
Organizers: Mr Robert Arnott and Dr Daphne Christie

Beyond the asylum: Anti-psychiatry and care in the community
Organizers: Dr Mark Jackson and Dr Daphne Christie

The Rhesus factor and disease prevention
Organizers: Professor Doris Zallen and Dr Daphne Christie

Platelets in thrombosis and other disorders
Organizers: Professor Gustav Born and Dr Daphne Christie

2004 **Short-course chemotherapy for tuberculosis**
Organizers: Dr Owen McCarthy and Dr Daphne Christie

Prenatal corticosteroids for reducing morbidity and mortality associated with preterm birth
Organizers: Sir Iain Chalmers and Dr Daphne Christie

Public health in the 1980s and 1990s: Decline and rise?
Organizers: Professor Virginia Berridge, Dr Niki Ellis and Dr Daphne Christie

2005 **The history of cholesterol, atherosclerosis and coronary disease**
Organizers: Professor Michael Oliver and Dr Daphne Christie

Development of physics applied to medicine in the UK, 1945–90
Organizers: Professor John Clifton and Dr Daphne Christie

PUBLISHED MEETINGS

"...Few books are so intellectually stimulating or uplifting".
Journal of the Royal Society of Medicine (1999) **92:** 206–8,
review of vols 1 and 2

"...This is oral history at its best...all the volumes make compulsive reading...they are, primarily, important historical records".
British Medical Journal (2002) **325**: 1119, review of the series

Technology transfer in Britain: The case of monoclonal antibodies
Self and non-self: A history of autoimmunity
Endogenous opiates
The Committee on Safety of Drugs
In: Tansey E M, Catterall P P, Christie D A, Willhoft S V, Reynolds L A. (eds) (1997) *Wellcome Witnesses to Twentieth Century Medicine.* Volume 1. London: The Wellcome Trust, 135pp. ISBN 1 869835 79 4

Making the human body transparent: The impact of NMR and MRI
Research in general practice
Drugs in psychiatric practice
The MRC Common Cold Unit
In: Tansey E M, Christie D A, Reynolds L A. (eds) (1998) *Wellcome Witnesses to Twentieth Century Medicine.* Volume 2. London: The Wellcome Trust, 282pp. ISBN 1 869835 39 5

Early heart transplant surgery in the UK
In: Tansey E M, Reynolds L A. (eds) (1999) *Wellcome Witnesses to Twentieth Century Medicine.* Volume 3. London: The Wellcome Trust, 72pp. ISBN 1 841290 07 6

Haemophilia: Recent history of clinical management
In: Tansey E M, Christie D A. (eds) (1999) *Wellcome Witnesses to Twentieth Century Medicine.* Volume 4. London: The Wellcome Trust, 90pp. ISBN 1 841290 08 4

Looking at the unborn: Historical aspects of obstetric ultrasound
In: Tansey E M, Christie D A. (eds) (2000) *Wellcome Witnesses to Twentieth*

Century Medicine. Volume 5. London: The Wellcome Trust, 80pp.
ISBN 1 841290 11 4

Post penicillin antibiotics: From acceptance to resistance?
In: Tansey E M, Reynolds L A. (eds) (2000) *Wellcome Witnesses to Twentieth Century Medicine*. Volume 6. London: The Wellcome Trust, 71pp.
ISBN 1 841290 12 2

Clinical research in Britain, 1950–1980
In: Reynolds L A, Tansey E M. (eds) (2000) *Wellcome Witnesses to Twentieth Century Medicine*. Volume 7. London: The Wellcome Trust, 74pp.
ISBN 1 841290 16 5

Intestinal absorption
In: Christie D A, Tansey E M. (eds) (2000) *Wellcome Witnesses to Twentieth Century Medicine*. Volume 8. London: The Wellcome Trust, 81pp.
ISBN 1 841290 17 3

Neonatal intensive care
In: Christie D A, Tansey E M. (eds) (2001) *Wellcome Witnesses to Twentieth Century Medicine*. Volume 9. London: The Wellcome Trust Centre for the History of Medicine at UCL, 84pp. ISBN 0 854840 76 1

British contributions to medical research and education in Africa after the Second World War
In: Reynolds L A, Tansey E M. (eds) (2001) *Wellcome Witnesses to Twentieth Century Medicine*. Volume 10. London: The Wellcome Trust Centre for the History of Medicine at UCL, 93pp. ISBN 0 854840 77 X

Childhood asthma and beyond
In: Reynolds L A, Tansey E M. (eds) (2001) *Wellcome Witnesses to Twentieth Century Medicine*. Volume 11. London: The Wellcome Trust Centre for the History of Medicine at UCL, 74pp. ISBN 0 854840 78 8

Maternal care
In: Christie D A, Tansey E M. (eds) (2001) *Wellcome Witnesses to Twentieth Century Medicine*. Volume 12. London: The Wellcome Trust Centre for the History of Medicine at UCL, 88pp. ISBN 0 854840 79 6

Population-based research in south Wales: The MRC Pneumoconiosis Research Unit and the MRC Epidemiology Unit
In: Ness A R, Reynolds L A, Tansey E M. (eds) (2002) *Wellcome Witnesses to Twentieth Century Medicine*. Volume 13. London: The Wellcome Trust Centre for the History of Medicine at UCL, 74pp. ISBN 0 854840 81 8

Peptic ulcer: Rise and fall
In: Christie D A, Tansey E M. (eds) (2002) *Wellcome Witnesses to Twentieth Century Medicine*. Volume 14. London: The Wellcome Trust Centre for the History of Medicine at UCL, 143pp. ISBN 0 854840 84 2

Leukaemia
In: Christie D A, Tansey E M. (eds) (2003) *Wellcome Witnesses to Twentieth Century Medicine*. Volume 15. London: The Wellcome Trust Centre for the History of Medicine at UCL, 86pp. ISBN 0 85484 087 7

The MRC Applied Psychology Unit
In: Reynolds L A, Tansey E M. (eds) (2003) *Wellcome Witnesses to Twentieth Century Medicine*. Volume 16. London: The Wellcome Trust Centre for the History of Medicine at UCL, 94pp. ISBN 0 85484 088 5

Genetic testing
In: Christie D A, Tansey E M. (eds) (2003) *Wellcome Witnesses to Twentieth Century Medicine*. Volume 17. London: The Wellcome Trust Centre for the History of Medicine at UCL, 130pp. ISBN 0 85484 094 X

Foot and mouth disease: The 1967 outbreak and its aftermath
In: Reynolds L A, Tansey E M. (eds) (2003) *Wellcome Witnesses to Twentieth Century Medicine*. Volume 18. London: The Wellcome Trust Centre for the History of Medicine at UCL, 114pp. ISBN 0 85484 096 6

Environmental toxicology: The legacy of *Silent Spring*
In: Christie D A, Tansey E M. (eds) (2004) *Wellcome Witnesses to Twentieth Century Medicine*. Volume 19. London: The Wellcome Trust Centre for the History of Medicine at UCL, 132pp. ISBN 0 85484 091 5

Cystic fibrosis
In: Christie D A, Tansey E M. (eds) (2004) *Wellcome Witnesses to Twentieth Century Medicine*. Volume 20. London: The Wellcome Trust Centre for the History of Medicine at UCL, 120pp. ISBN 0 85484 086 9

Innovation in pain management
In: Reynolds L A, Tansey E M. (eds) (2004) *Wellcome Witnesses to Twentieth Century Medicine.* Volume 21. London: The Wellcome Trust Centre for the History of Medicine at UCL, 125pp. ISBN 0 85484 097 4

The Rhesus factor and disease prevention
In: Zallen D T, Christie D A, Tansey E M. (eds) (2004) *Wellcome Witnesses to Twentieth Century Medicine.* Volume 22. London: The Wellcome Trust Centre for the History of Medicine at UCL, 98pp. ISBN 0 85484 099 0

The recent history of platelets in thrombosis and other disorders
In: Reynolds L A, Tansey E M. (eds) (2005) *Wellcome Witnesses to Twentieth Century Medicine.* Volume 23. London: The Wellcome Trust Centre for the History of Medicine at UCL, this volume. ISBN 0 85484 103 2

Short-course chemotherapy for tuberculosis
In: Christie D A, Tansey E M. (eds) (2005) *Wellcome Witnesses to Twentieth Century Medicine.* Volume 24. London: The Wellcome Trust Centre for the History of Medicine at UCL, 120pp. ISBN 0 85484 104 0

Prenatal corticosteroids for reducing morbidity and mortality associated with preterm birth
In: Reynolds L A, Tansey E M. (eds) (2005) *Wellcome Witnesses to Twentieth Century Medicine.* Volume 25. London: The Wellcome Trust Centre for the History of Medicine at UCL. In press.

Public health in the 1980s and 1990s: Decline and rise?
In: Berridge V, Christie D A, Tansey E M. (eds) (2005) *Wellcome Witnesses to Twentieth Century Medicine.* Volume 26. London: The Wellcome Trust Centre for the History of Medicine at UCL. In press.

Volumes 1–12 cost £5 plus postage, with volumes 13–20 at £10 each. Orders of four or more volumes receive a 20 per cent discount. All 20 published volumes in the series are available at the special price of £115 plus postage. To order a copy contact t.tillotson@wellcome.ac.uk or by phone: +44 (0)20 7611 8486; or fax: +44 (0)20 7611 8703.

All volumes are freely available online under publications at www.ucl.ac.uk/histmed
A hard copy of volumes 21–24 can be ordered from www.amazon.co.uk; www.amazon.com; and all good booksellers.

Other publications

Technology transfer in Britain: The case of monoclonal antibodies
In: Tansey E M, Catterall P P. (1993) *Contemporary Record* **9**: 409–44.

Monoclonal antibodies: A witness seminar on contemporary medical history
In: Tansey E M, Catterall P P. (1994) *Medical History* **38**: 322–7.

Chronic pulmonary disease in South Wales coalmines: An eye-witness account of the MRC surveys (1937–42)
In: P D'Arcy Hart, edited and annotated by E M Tansey. (1998) *Social History of Medicine* **11**: 459–68.

Ashes to Ashes – The history of smoking and health
In: Lock S P, Reynolds L A, Tansey E M. (eds) (1998) Amsterdam: Rodopi BV, 228pp. ISBN 90420 0396 0 (Hfl 125) (hardback). Reprinted 2003.

Witnessing medical history. An interview with Dr Rosemary Biggs
Professor Christine Lee and Dr Charles Rizza (interviewers). (1998) *Haemophilia* **4**: 769–77.

Witnessing the Witnesses: Pitfalls and potentials of the Witness Seminar in twentieth century medicine
By E M Tansey. In: Doel R, Soderqvist T. (eds) (2005) *Writing Recent Science: The historiography of contemporary science, technology and medicine.* London: Routledge.

INTRODUCTION

We had hoped that this introduction would be written by John Vane. Sadly, he died in November 2004 after a prolonged illness. His enormous contributions to the field of prostaglandins, and their influences in platelet behaviour, were referred to many times during the meeting and were very much in everyone's minds throughout it.

An interesting account of the early recognition of platelets in thrombosis is given by the late John French in his chapter on thrombosis in Florey's *General Pathology* – a wonderful book with a star-studded cast of authors that Lord Florey gathered around him in the Sir William Dunn School of Pathology in Oxford. French recounts how in 1851 Wharton-Jones described an artery becoming blocked 'by a mass composed apparently of colourless corpuscles and fibrin'.[1] In 1875, Zahn (who described the lines of platelets in thrombi that bear his name) observed cells deposited on the inner wall of a vessel injured by pressure or salt. However, both Wharton-Jones and Zahn mistook the cells for leukocytes, since the platelets in frog's blood have nuclei. It was thought that what were in fact non-nucleated mammalian platelets were simply cell fragments not normally present in the circulation. In 1882, Bizzozero repeated Zahn's experiment, this time using guinea-pigs or young rabbits, whose platelets are non-nucleated. Recognition of platelets as one of the cellular elements of blood was therefore established, along with their potential for being 'agglutinated' and stabilized at sites of injury.

The modern era of platelet research started with the introduction of *ex vivo* methods for studying platelet behaviour. Helen Payling Wright developed her technique for assessing platelet adhesiveness to glass.[2] However, it was of course the introduction of the platelet aggregometer by Gustav Born, described in 1962, that marks the beginning of the detailed study of the way platelets behave and respond to various stimuli, and that is where the proceedings of this meeting really start.[3] There is no doubt whatever about the role of platelets in thrombosis and in clinically manifest vascular disease, not only heart attacks and strokes but also in venous thrombosis. The

[1] French (1958): 185.

[2] Wright (1941).

[3] Born (1962b). See also Smith (2004).

demonstration that aspirin reduces platelet aggregability led to an enormous number of laboratory and clinical studies on its value and also to a series of randomized controlled trials that have shown its great value in both the primary and secondary prevention of thrombotic disorders. John Vane's elucidation of the effects of aspirin on prostaglandins, for which he won the Nobel Prize,[4] opened up a new direction for studies that have – among many other things – enabled rational decisions about aspirin dosage to be made.

We know a great deal about the biochemistry and physiology of platelets and how to modify them to good effect. It remains a paradox that we still lack a validated test for clinical use to identify those whose thrombotic episodes are due to the sensitivity or activity of their platelets. Maybe this no longer matters! Anyway, these proceedings will I hope raise questions for future endeavours in the platelet field as well as presenting an interesting and authoritative account of its recent history.

Tom Meade

London School of Hygiene and Tropical Medicine

[4] Vane (1971, 1983).

THE RECENT HISTORY OF PLATELETS IN THROMBOSIS AND OTHER DISORDERS

The transcript of a Witness Seminar held by the Wellcome Trust Centre for the History of Medicine at UCL, London, on 25 November 2003

Edited by L A Reynolds and E M Tansey

THE RECENT HISTORY OF PLATELETS IN THROMBOSIS AND OTHER DISORDERS

Participants

Dr Y S [Mick] Bakhle
Professor Sir Christopher Booth
Professor Gustav Born
Professor Donald Chambers
Professor John Dickinson
Professor Peter Elwood
Professor Rod Flower
Professor Alison Goodall
Professor John Hampton
Professor Michael Harrison
Professor Stan Heptinstall
Dr Peter Hunter
Dr Peter MacCallum
Dr Martyn Mahaut-Smith
Professor Tom Meade (Chair)
Professor Salvador Moncada
Professor Michael Oliver
Professor Clive Page
Professor Sir Stanley Peart
Professor Colin Prentice
Professor Peter Richardson
Dr Stewart Sage
Dr Tilli Tansey
Dr Duncan Thomas

Among those attending the meeting: Dr Valerie Alabaster, Dr Nicky Begent, Mr Andrew Beswick, Dr Joseph Blau, Dr Jack Botting, Dr Renia Botting, Dr Richard Farndale, Dr Richard Jarvis, Dr Kiheung Kim, Professor Jeremy Pearson, Mr Ian Roney, Dr Pia Siljander, Mrs Felicity Youlten, Dr Lawrence Youlten

Apologies include: Professor Sir Charles George, Dr John Gordon, Professor Susanna Hourani, Dr Michael Humphreys, Professor John Martin, Professor Carlo Patrono, Professor Sir John Vane,* Dr Steve Watson, Dr Harvey Weiss

* Died 19 November 2004

'THROMBOLYSIS' WITNESS SEMINAR PARTICIPANTS†

Dr Hewan Dewar
Professor Sir Richard Doll
Professor John Hampton
Dr Arthur Hollman
Professor Desmond Julian
Dr Robin Norris
Professor Brian Pentecost (Chair)
Professor Tom Quinn
Dr Roger Smith
Professor Andrew Stevens

† Edited and annotated extract from the Witness Seminar, 'Thrombolysis', held by the Wellcome Trust Centre for the History of Medicine at UCL, London, on 28 January 2003, which appears as Appendix 3, on pages 93–112.

Dr Tilli Tansey: This meeting was suggested by Professor Gustav Born and was agreed to by the Programme Committee, and we are very grateful to him for suggesting such an interesting topic. My colleague Daphne Christie has worked very closely with Professor Born and with Professor Meade in organizing this meeting, and I would like to thank them all for that work. It's very important to identify a suitable chairman for these meetings, someone who knows the subject and who is going to be able to keep control of all the participants. I am delighted that Tom Meade has agreed to chair this meeting and so without further ado we will hand over to Tom.

Professor Tom Meade:[1] Welcome to this meeting, which I think will certainly be extremely interesting. There are several topics that we should address, though obviously there will be quite a lot of overlap between different aspects. After I have asked Gustav Born and Stan Heptinstall to introduce their topic and after we have had some discussion about that, I shall say a few words about platelets and the prediction of thrombotic disorders.[2] I will ask Duncan Thomas and Clive Page to follow and that will take us up to tea. After tea we will start off with Rod Flower. And, Salvador Moncada (who has just come at very short notice, for which we are most grateful), obviously we would like you to say something about the historical aspects of the prostaglandin story.

We will start off with Gustav Born who is, of course, the person most associated in many ways with the whole platelet story. As to the clinical side of things, I suggest we stick to coronary heart disease and stroke, but that is only a suggestion. Obviously, aspirin with its effects on platelets has now been implicated in a number of other conditions – perhaps large bowel cancer is the one that is attracting most attention at the moment, but let's not stray too far from platelets. So, Gus, would you like to start off by introducing the question of platelets, aggregometry and biochemical aspects.

Professor Gustav Born: In my work on platelets, I have enjoyed the collaboration and friendship of more than 40 co-workers from this and many other countries. They and our publications are listed and our work is summarized in the 'Afterword', which I was invited to contribute to the 1000-page tome on *Platelets* in 2002.[3] What follows is a selection from research on platelets and other circulatory topics done from the 1960s to the 1980s.

[1] Biographical notes appear on pages 145–56.

[2] For details on the discovery of platelets, see Robb-Smith (1967).

[3] Professor Gustav Born based his introductory remarks on 'Afterword: Platelets, a personal story' in Gresele *et al.* (2002): 1063–71.

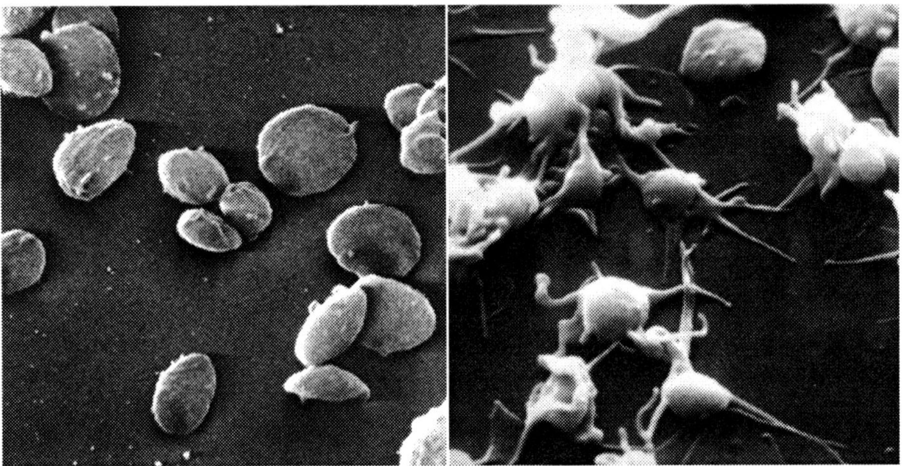

Figure 1: (Above left) Scanning electron micrograph of platelets [x 15 000], *c*. 1965.
Figure 2: (Above right) Scanning electron micrograph of aggregated platelets [x 15 000], *c*. 1965.

During that period descriptive knowledge of platelets was superseded by understanding of their pathophysiological mechanisms and functions.

How does one come to platelets? The most common route has been through clinical haematology; and until platelets became prominent players in coronary heart disease and stroke, their medical importance was mainly *in absentia*, because platelet deficiency causes bleeding. There are many causes of platelet deficiency, one being radiation. As an Army Medical Officer posted close to atom-bombed Hiroshima in defeated Japan after the Second World War, deadly haemorrhages from radiation sickness first made me aware of platelets and how much we need them.

My own long-term relationship with platelets came through postdoctoral initiation into pharmacological research. In 1956 I was working in the Oxford Pharmacology Department with Hugh Blaschko on the recently discovered association of adrenaline with adenosine triphosphate (ATP) in adrenal granules, which contain about three molecules of the cationic amine for each molecule of ATP^{3-}, suggesting ionic binding.[4] It occurred to me that other endogenous amines might be stored similarly elsewhere in the body. I had heard or read of platelets containing large amounts of the vasoconstrictor amine serotonin (5-hydroxytryptamine, 5-HT). So the initial intention was to

[4] Blaschko *et al.* (1956).

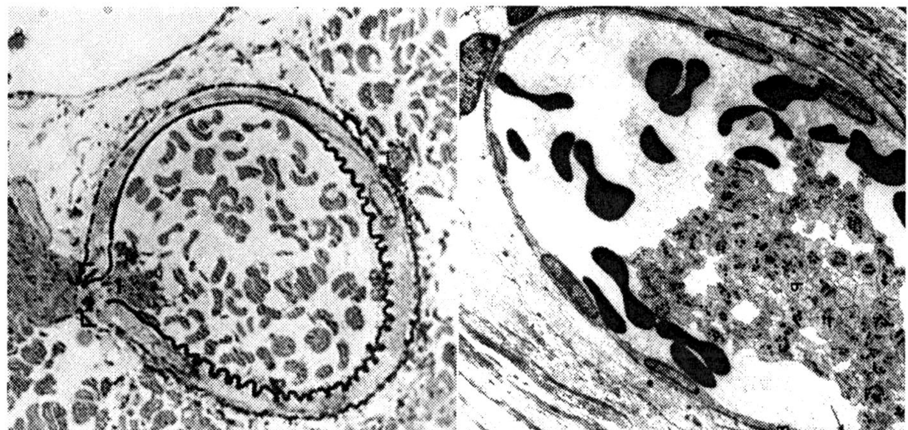

Figure 3: (Above left) Platelets aggregating as a 'haemostatic plug' [x 650].
Figure 4: (Above right) Platelets aggregating as an intravascular thrombus [x 3000].

utilize this circulating pseudocell [platelet] for pharmacological purposes. I was the first person in Britain to use the firefly luminescence method, recently introduced by McElroy in the US, for measuring ATP.[5] With the platelet extract adjusted to ATP concentrations expected from other cell types, the galvanometer pointer flew off the scale – an unforgettable moment.[6] The discovery of excess platelet ATP was indeed followed by evidence for its stoichiometric association with 5-HT, again suggesting ionic binding.

By far the largest and most enduring part of my work on platelets had to do with their role in haemostasis and thrombosis, both the physiological and the pathological processes that happen through aggregation of the platelets. My interest in platelet aggregation was awakened by the coming together of two previously unconnected observations. One was our discovery of excess ATP in platelets and the demonstration of its rapid breakdown in clotting blood.[7] The other was the Norwegians' discovery of the platelet-aggregating effect of adenosine diphosphate (ADP).[8] By then we were aware that the primary function of platelets is their haemostatic aggregation. I suggested that the two

[5] Strehler and Totter (1954).

[6] Born (1956a).

[7] Born (1956b).

[8] Gaarder *et al.* (1961).

processes are connected through the formation of ADP from ATP released from platelets and from other cells involved in vascular injury.[9] Nevertheless, over the years the hypothesis that ADP contributes to platelet aggregation in haemostasis and thrombosis has been supported by experiments and by clinical trials of drugs which inhibit platelet activation by ADP, notably the 'Clopidogrel versus Aspirin in Patients at Risk of Ischaemic Events' (CAPRIE) trial published in the *Lancet* as recently as 1996.[10]

For investigations of platelet physiology I invented and developed the optical aggregometer for quantifying and analysing platelet reactions *in vitro*. The idea came to me from so-called 'turbidimetric' measurements of ribonuclease activity in *Streptomyces* culture filtrates that I had done for my DPhil in Oxford. I made the simple adaptations appropriate for measuring platelet aggregation in plasma. The method is simple, indeed quite banal, and nothing to be proud of intellectually.[11] But it became an amazing success, by bringing exciting results quickly and reproducibly. Having had an important part of my scientific upbringing in Professor Harold Burn's excellent Pharmacology Department in Oxford, where free and noisy communication between members and visitors was strongly encouraged, I had no hesitation in demonstrating the technique immediately to anybody who asked.[12] The method was published in 1962[13] and the first detailed description of observations made with it appeared in the following year.[14] We quantified the relation of aggregate formation to the optical changes[15] and showed that they could be accounted for by classical light-scattering theory.[16]

---

[9] Professor Gustav Born wrote: 'This has turned out to be an oversimplification as far as the platelets themselves are concerned, which release ADP mostly from a different pool than that in which ATP breaks down. The evidence is that ADP and thromboxane A_2 contribute about equally to haemostatic aggregation *in vivo*.' Note on draft transcript, 25 February 2005. Born (1962b).

[10] CAPRIE (1996).

[11] Optical aggregometry is a technique to measure platelet aggregation, where a platelet agonist such as adrenaline, ADP or collagen is added to platelet-rich plasma to induce aggregation. See Figure 5. The most easily interpreted measurement is the initial velocity of increase in light. Results vary according to the platelet count and agonist used. See page 27 for its use to investigate the pharmacology of a single human cell type.

[12] A letter from Sir John Vane, 2 May 2001, on this subject has been deposited along with the records of this meeting in GC/253, Archives and Manuscripts, Wellcome Library, London.

[13] Born (1962a and b).

[14] Born and Cross (1963b).

[15] Born and Hume (1967); Michal and Born (1971).

[16] Latimer *et al.* (1977).

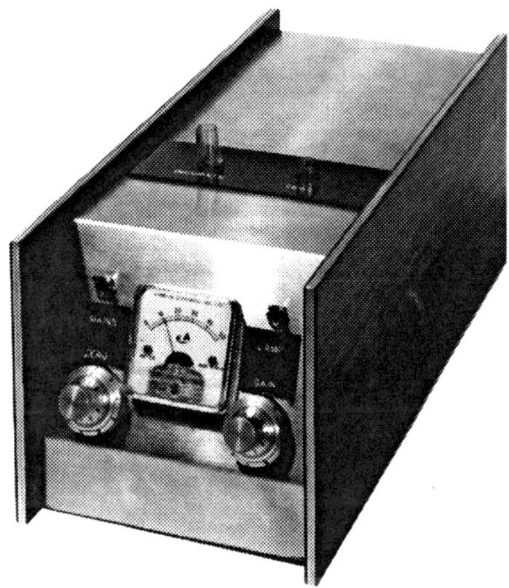

Figure 5: The first aggregometer made in the workshop at the Royal College of Surgeons in 1961. Born (1962b).

The optical aggregometer has ever since been used worldwide in fundamental, clinical and epidemiological investigations.[17] Within a few years the original papers became Citation Classics,[18] and by January 2001 the *Nature* paper had been cited 3796 times and the *Journal of Physiology* paper 1902 times. (This information is from Peter Richardson.)[19] Many more papers, probably thousands, have been based on optical aggregometry without reference to the original publications.[20]

---

[17] Among those who have manufactured Born aggregometers commercially are Alpha Laboratories, Eastleigh, Hants, UK; H Upchurch & Co., Leicester, UK; Entec GmbH, Ilmenau, Germany; Bryston Manufacturing Limited, Rexdale, Ontario, Canada; Payton Associates, Scarborough, Ontario, Canada; and Payton Scientific, Inc., Buffalo, NY; Bio/Data Corp., Horsham, PA; Chrono-log, Havertown, PA; and Sienco Inc., Morrison, CO.

[18] A Citation Classic is a frequently cited article chosen by *Science Citation Index,* a journal that first appeared in 1963, as among the top most frequently cited articles, featuring a commentary on its influence and a facsimile of the article, freely available at www.garfield.library.upenn.edu/classics.html (visited 15 April 2005) and published in *Current Contents;* for an essay on citation indexing, see http://garfield.library.upenn.edu/essays/V1p158y1962-73.pdf (visited 15 April 2005). See also Born (1977, 1989).

[19] Professor Gustav Born wrote: 'In 2004 the latter was the sixth most cited paper ever published in the *Journal* (this information is from Stewart Sage, the Editor).' Note on draft transcript, 25 February 2005.

[20] Professor Gustav Born suggested three possible reasons that this paper is one of the most cited articles ever published, see Gresele *et al.* (2002): 1065–6.

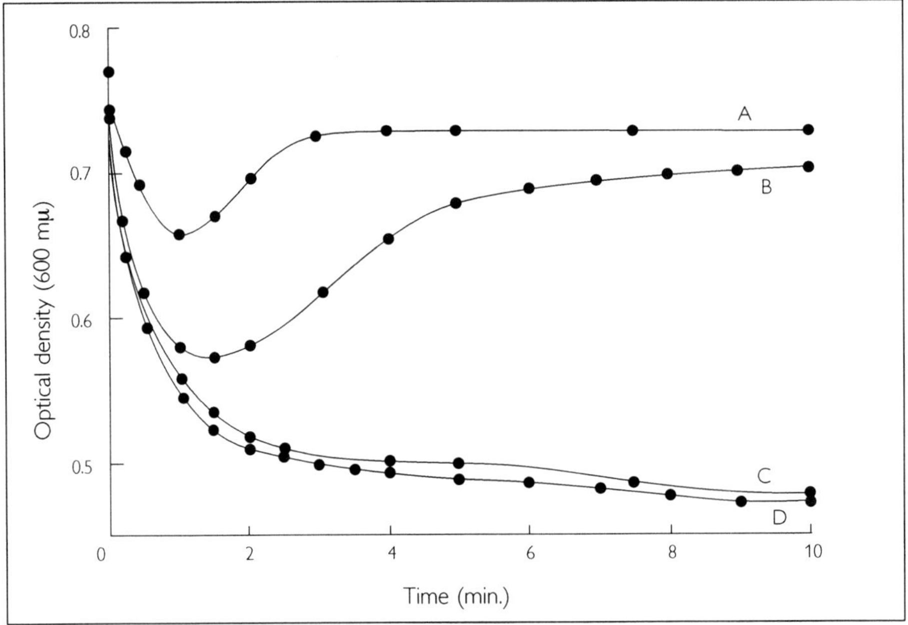

Figure 6: The first optical record of platelet aggregation by ADP showing the increase in transmitted light, illustrated here as downward deflection.

Different concentrations of ADP was added at time O: (A) 2.5 x 10^{-7} M; (B) 5 x 10^{-7} M; (C) 1 x 10^{-6} M; (D) 2.5 x 10^{-6} M.

Born (1962b).

I have been told that there are thousands of optical aggregometers around the world, and am often asked why I did not patent the device. The reason I give is that before the Thatcherite degradation of everything in life to money, it did not occur to me, nor to most members of the medical research community, to patent inventions or discoveries; indeed my Oxford Professor, Howard Florey, was against patenting anything of potential medical value.[21] So the idea just never came up.

Up to the molecular biology era it is probably true to say that much if not most of the new information about platelets has depended on optical aggregometry.[22] We characterized aggregation with respect to velocity and temperature and pH dependence, and discovered two essential cofactors of aggregation, namely calcium and fibrinogen;[23] and the suggestion that fibrinogen formed 'bridges'

[21] See Macfarlane (1979). For further discussion about patents, see, for example, http://biotech.about.com/library/weekly/aa_penicillinpatent.htm (visited 14 October 2004).

[22] See note 11.

[23] Born and Cross (1964); Cross (1964).

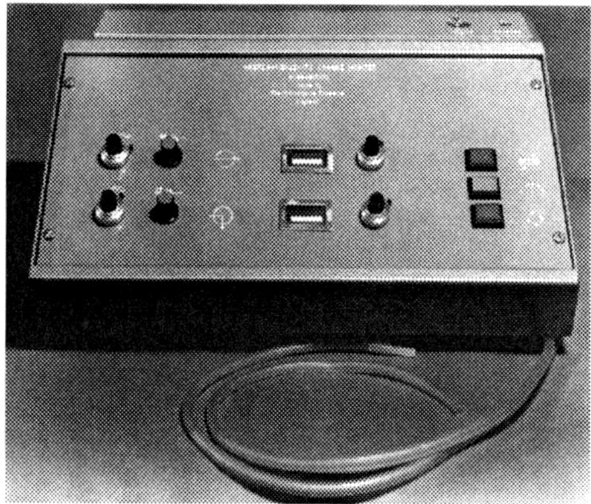

Figure 7: A modern single-channel aggregometer, 1970.

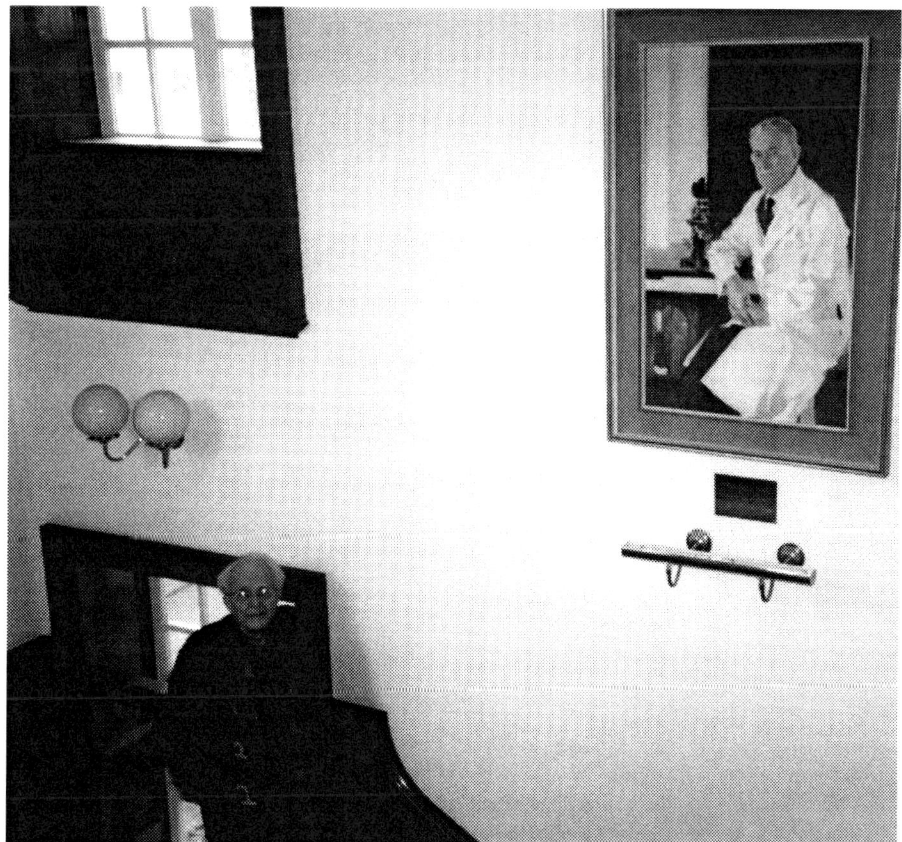

Figure 8: Professor Gustav Born standing near the portrait of Lord Florey at the Dunn School of Pathology at Oxford, 2004.

linking aggregating platelets was later confirmed at the electron microscopic and molecular levels.[24]

The rapid shape change of platelets (time constant of about 1 second at 37°C), the first visual evidence of their activation, was quantified and shown to conform to Michaelis–Menten kinetics.[25] The results suggested that aggregation agonists such as ADP react with specific membrane receptors leading to structural changes. Now, of course, these receptors are fully identified.[26]

Optical aggregometry made possible the discovery by Macmillan and Oliver in 1965 of the second phase of aggregation[27] – Michael Cross and I had failed to notice, or to think about, the anomalous deformations in our manually plotted aggregometer tracings (this was before the availability of continuous recording), which turned out to be the optical manifestation of the platelet release reaction.[28] It is this second phase of aggregation that is inhibited by aspirin.[29] Therefore optical aggregometry is at the beginning of a very important medical story.

Optical aggregometry soon led also to our discovery of the first aggregation inhibitors, namely ATP and adenosine, looked at first because of their close chemical relationship to proaggregatory ADP.[30]

---

[24] Professor Gustav Born wrote: 'Nowadays this bridging function, and thereby platelet aggregation, can be prevented by various molecules which inhibit binding of fibrinogen to its receptor, the activated conformer of glycoprotein IIb-IIIa, on the platelet surface.' Note on draft transcript, 25 February 2005. Born (1965).

[25] Born (1970).

[26] Professor Gustav Born wrote: 'The shape change paper [note 25] also contains the proof, by means of a novel thrombocrit technique for determining cell volume directly, that the rapid shape change is not accompanied by an increase in mean platelet volume, as had been widely accepted on the basis of Coulter Counter measurements. Such a rapid increase in cell volume would, to my knowledge, be unique in cell biology and indeed impossible because of cell lysis.' Note on draft transcript, 25 February 2005.

[27] Macmillan and Oliver (1965).

[28] Professor Gustav Born wrote: 'In this reaction, enough ADP is released (and thromboxane A_2 formed) to account for the positive feedback mechanism of aggregation proposed earlier.' Note on draft transcript, 25 February 2005. See Figure 14 and note 162.

[29] See note 27.

[30] Born (1962b); Clayton *et al.* (1963).

As it has turned out, inhibition was the most exciting and far-reaching discovery because it established the therapeutic possibility of preventing arterial thrombosis by means of antiplatelet drugs and initiated the era of their use for the prevention of myocardial infarction (MI) and stroke. We devoted much effort to inhibitory mechanisms. To demonstrate this rigorously required correlating optical aggregometry with quantitative electron microscopy.[31]

For quantifying aggregation *in vivo*, novel techniques were developed for reproducible bleeding time determinations from small arteries in the superior mesenteric territory of rats and rabbits. In both species local infusions of active but not of inactive ADP-removing enzyme systems increased bleeding time significantly, supporting the conclusion that platelet aggregation in primary haemostasis involves ADP.[32] In rats these bleeding times were also prolonged by ADP receptor antagonists.[33] This work was done, incidentally, with a great-granddaughter of Charles Darwin, Carola, a charming girl. With ultra-sensitive luminescence measurements, blood at arterial puncture sites was shown to contain micromolar ATP for at least two or three seconds.[34] Its rapid dephosphorylation supported the proposition[35] that ADP is involved in initiating the haemostatic aggregation.[36]

Quantifying platelet adhesiveness and aggregation in uninjured vessels required a further methodological innovation. This was to apply ADP by micro-iontophoresis to the outsides of small blood vessels.[37] ADP thus applied showed that platelet thrombi can be made to form many times on the same site without damaging the endothelial lining, thereby disposing of claims to the contrary. Aggregates grew exponentially, the rate constant providing a measure of the effects of blood flow and of inhibitors.[38] The technique also permitted a

---

[31] Professor Gustav Born wrote: 'We did, *inter alia*, experiments on ourselves which could conceivably have been harmful and would now be strictly forbidden. These showed that the relative potency of adenosine analogues as aggregation inhibitors and as arterial vasodilators was the same. Born *et al.* (1965). See also Born *et al.* (1978).

[32] Zawilska *et al.* (1982); Begent and Born (1983).

[33] Born *et al.* (1986)

[34] Born and Kratzer (1984); Kratzer and Born (1985).

[35] Born (1962a).

[36] Born (1962b).

[37] Duling *et al.* (1968).

[38] Begent and Born (1970).

first determination of platelet activation time (of the order of 100 milliseconds, since revised downwards).[39]

As it has turned out, the demonstration that inhibitors of *in vitro* aggregation are also effective *in vivo* has been of great importance. Regional administration of aggregation inhibitors prevented thrombosis formation in artificial organs, work done with Peter Richardson.[40]

For platelet people, the most important discoveries in the 1970s were proaggregatory thromboxane A_2 produced by platelets and antiaggregatory prostacyclin produced by vessel walls; and of course the Nobel Prize-winning discovery by John Vane of the action of aspirin in inhibiting prostaglandin biosynthesis,[41] plus the immediate demonstration of its applicability to platelets by our graduate students Bryan Smith and Jim Willis.[42]

Looking back,[43] I suppose that the greatest change to have happened to platelets is their enormously increased importance in clinical medicine – from somehow being involved in the rather uncommon conditions of idiopathic thrombocytopaenia and radiation sickness to being recognized as a dominant factor in arterial thromboses causing MI and stroke, which together cause

---

[39] Born and Richardson (1980).

[40] Richardson *et al.* (1976).

[41] Professor Gustav Born wrote: 'These events are very well known, and the therapeutic advances they brought are very great: through its antiplatelet action aspirin reduces the risk of heart attacks and strokes by up to 40 per cent. This prostaglandin period also renewed interest in the influence of diet on platelet thrombogenesis, which Dick Philip and I had shown some years before to be accelerated in fat-fed rats [Born and Philip (1965)]. In the early 1980s Margareta Thorngren and I produced human evidence that a fish diet of a month did not diminish platelet-derived thromboxane A_2 in bleeding time blood, and that the increased haemorrhagic tendency of fish-eating populations has less to do with platelets than with vascular contractility – at a time a heretical proposition which has presumably been confirmed since [Begent *et al.* (1984)].' Note on draft transcript, 25 February 2005.

[42] Vane (1971); Smith and Willis (1971); Ferreira *et al.* (1971). See also, Willis and Smith (1981); for a description of Vane's reasoning on the action of aspirin, see Vane (1992).

[43] Professor Gustav Born wrote: 'By the mid-1980s understanding of the physiological behaviour and pharmacological control of platelets was well advanced. New questions were increasingly answered by the techniques of molecular biology, with which I was not familiar. So it seemed natural to devote my last research decade to atherosclerosis, the more so because to the extent that it will become preventable, the clinical importance of arterial thrombosis and therewith of platelets will diminish. These contributions have been reviewed [Born *et al.* (2003)].' Note on draft transcript, 25 February 2005.

almost half the deaths in industrialized populations. It is gratifying that the feedback hypothesis of platelet aggregation turned out to be the explanation of the remarkable effectiveness of antiplatelet drugs of the aspirin type in the prevention of heart attacks and strokes.

Platelet research has been continuously interesting in itself, and it has also permitted following promising side alleys.[44] I am glad to have contributed in a small way to knowledge of a vital physiological process – haemostasis – and to an advance in medicine, which Dr Samuel Johnson rightly called the greatest benefit to mankind.[45]

Meade: There's obviously a lot there that we will want to come back to, but I will now ask Stan Heptinstall to say a few words on the same subject.

Professor Stan Heptinstall: I am sorry that I am here, in one sense, in that I am not old enough. I look around and I see people whom for the whole of my career I have thought of as my seniors. I didn't come on the scene until 1972. I went from Newcastle to Nottingham to work with Tony Mitchell [see Figure 9] on an Medical Research Council (MRC) programme grant. There was a guy there before me called David Nichols, but he was a mitochondriologist and he soon discovered that platelets didn't have many mitochondria, so he saw the light and went off somewhere else. I answered the advert that resulted from his departure. Then I started to meet the people that I see today in this room.

I don't think I have really done very much in my career. When I started to work on platelets, a lot of what Gustav has just been talking about had already been described. We knew that platelets aggregated. We knew that ADP and a long, long list of other things induced aggregation. John Hampton discovered that noradrenaline aggregated platelets. John and I worked together with Tony Mitchell in Nottingham. I remember looking at a table in a publication by Fraser Mustard – I think it was in *Pharmacological Reviews*, dated 1970.[46] It contained a long list of things that made platelets aggregate together. So we knew about aggregation, we knew about glycoprotein deficiencies, we knew about Glanzmann's thrombasthaenia, we knew about Bernard–Soulier

---

[44] Professor Gustav Born wrote: 'A totally unexpected, extraordinarily interesting development has been a continuing burst of research on trypanosomiasis, African sleeping sickness.' Note on draft transcript, 25 February 2005. See James and Born (1980); Born (2003b).

[45] Chantler (2002) questions whether medicine can still make this claim.

[46] Mustard and Packham (1970).

syndrome and so on. We knew that platelets underwent vicious metamorphosis. Later on, this became known as the release reaction. We knew that platelets were associated with bleeding problems as a consequence of glycoprotein deficiencies. We had a good idea that platelets were involved in thrombosis, and the idea was developing that agents that modulate platelet function, antiplatelet agents, might be used as antithrombotic agents. The whole of my career was based upon moving all of that forward

I like to think of myself as having been an enabler, as opposed to a discovering scientist. For example, getting involved in the grouping that Duncan Thomas and Colin Prentice put together following the International Society for Thrombosis and Haemostasis (ISTH) conference in the UK back in 1979, when the British Society for Haemostasis and Thrombosis came into existence in 1980.[47] Later on I became Secretary and then President of that society. A lot of the work that was performed by UK people was presented at the British Society of Haemostasis and Thrombosis meetings. I also feel that I have made an impact on the European dimension, because years ago, back in 1981, I went to the old East Germany (a really exciting thing to do at that time, to go behind the Iron Curtain) to meet people there. In collaboration with the people in Erfurt, East Germany, we set up a series of European conferences which people from the UK attended. These were successful, because they brought together people from eastern and western Europe. Latterly I became editor of the journal *Platelets.*

I have been asked to speak about aggregation. My first look at aggregation was at Nottingham. I didn't know what a platelet was. I just wanted to go and work on something relevant to physiology and/or disease, and platelets seemed to fit the bill. I was introduced to Gustav Born's equipment [the aggregometer], which in those days was nothing more than a stirring device and a galvanometer. The platelet-rich plasma was put in the stirring device and it was stirred for a bit. You didn't worry too much about temperature and every now and then you took it out and plunged it in the galvanometer to read the optical density. Then you plotted out the results. It's amazing what results could be obtained from such a crude system. I am not being disparaging at all to Gustav, but it was a crude system. A few years later, in collaboration with the late John Adams, who was a technician, and also Peter Jessop at the University of

---

[47] The inaugural meeting of the British Society for Haemostasis and Thrombosis was held in London in 1980, with Professor Gustav Born as the first President and Dr Duncan Thomas as the first Secretary. See www.bsht.bham.ac.uk/History.htm (visited 13 April 2005). For the background of the ISTH, see Glossary, page 163.

Nottingham, we built our own six-channel automated platelet aggregometer which was based upon the Born principle. We published that in 1975.[48] We used that machine for many years until we bought one of the more modern commercial instruments later on. And I have to say that even now Born aggregometry is the gold standard. There are other techniques that are available for measuring platelet aggregation, but Born aggregometry continues to be the gold standard. It is not perfect. It only measures what I like to call macroaggregation, that is the formation of large aggregates that can be seen by the naked eye.[49] It's at that point that the optical density of the sample starts to change. The technique tells you nothing about any microaggregation that may have occurred before that. Of course, using Born aggregometry, all you are getting is information on the ability of platelets to aggregate together in the absence of other blood cells, and it turns out that other blood cells are very important in determining what platelets do. But nevertheless, Born aggregometry remains the gold standard.

There are other techniques. I see Rod Flower, who developed the impedence aggregometer for measuring platelet aggregation in whole blood, which is still used today. It didn't take off to the same extent as Born aggregation, simply because you can't see the aggregates. You know, you can't see them visually. I think the beauty of Gustav's technique is that you can actually see the aggregates being generated.

In our own laboratories, we have done an enormous amount of work over the years in which we measured platelet aggregation using a platelet-counting technique. The concept is very simple. As platelets aggregate together, the number of single platelets in whole blood reduces, and therefore if you continually monitor the platelet count in the sample, you can get a very good estimate of the degree of aggregation that occurs. And if you use flow cytometry in conjunction with that, then you can very clearly see microaggregates being generated and you can look at the effects of the

---

[48] Adams *et al.* (1975).

[49] Professor Gustav Born wrote: 'Not so. See Born and Hume (1967).' Note on draft transcript, 25 February 2005. Professor Stan Heptinstall wrote: 'Well, even if this is not absolutely correct there there is still a huge difference between techniques that rely on light absorbance that can only detect macroaggregation and, for example, techniques that use platelet counting which detect microaggregation. With the latter you can see aggregation occurring in the early seconds following agonist addition at the time the light absorbance is still increasing consequent to shape change. See Fox *et al.* (2004).' E-mail to Mrs Lois Reynolds, 26 April 2005.

pharmacological agents and you can look at the effects of disease states and the differences that occur.

The other area I was asked to say something about is platelet biochemistry. Platelet biochemistry – signal transmission inside platelets – is an area that continues to develop. Someone finds out something new every week. It's an incredibly complex area. Back in the early 1970s, it was known that there were lots of agents that make platelets aggregate together. It was known that glycoproteins such as GPIIb/IIIa were involved. We were starting to get an inkling of the sorts of things that happened inside platelets, such as calcium mobilization. Stewart Sage over there, who's done an enormous amount of work on calcium mobilization in platelets and other cells, may well want to say something about the history of that later on. I remember people like Tim Rink being involved in developing the processes for measuring calcium mobilization.[50] Cyclic AMP was also important, of course.

This is very much a UK gathering, isn't it? However, a lot of UK people who have done an enormous amount of work on platelets have actually gone abroad to do it. Some who come to mind are people like Alan Nurton, Ken Clemetson, and John McGregor, who went to work in France, and Richard Haslam, who went to Canada and did a lot of work in the cyclic AMP area. I will miss lots and lots of people out in this very brief, off the top of my head, presentation. I really do apologize for that.

We knew a bit about calcium, we knew a bit about cyclic AMP. Shortly thereafter thromboxane A_2 was identified by Bengt Samuelsson.[51] I am sure Professor Moncada will put me right if I get anything wrong here. John Vane and, of course, Salvador Moncada, were very much involved in the aspirin story and the discovery of prostacyclin and the effects of nitric oxide (NO) on platelets.

What I would like to say is that I have had the privilege of working on platelets for over 31 years now, and I have thoroughly enjoyed it. I don't think I have personally made a big mark, but I have very much enjoyed watching what many of you in this room have done.

---

[50] See, for example, Rink *et al.* (1982); Rink (1982, 1987).

[51] Professor Bengt Samuelsson shared the 1982 Nobel Prize in Physiology or Medicine with Professor Sune Bergström and Professor Sir John Vane for their discoveries 'concerning prostaglandins and related biologically active substances'. See http://nobelprize.org/medicine/laureates/1982/index.html (visited 18 October 2004).

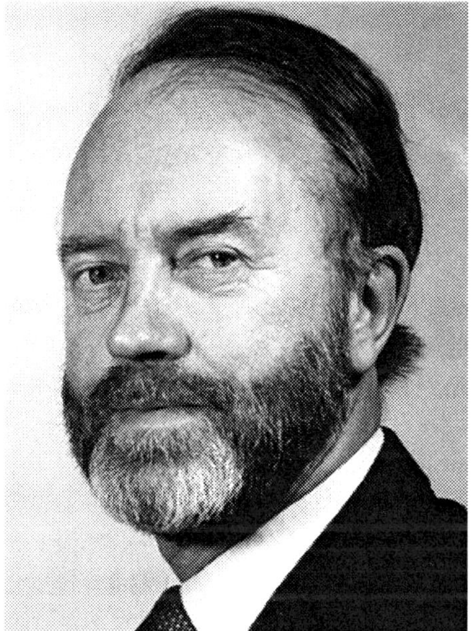
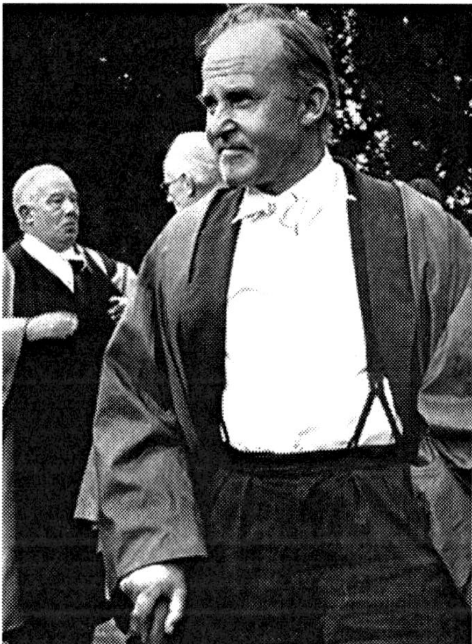

Figure 9 (left): Professor Tony Mitchell, *c.* 1960s.
Figure 10 (right): Professor Sir George Pickering at the Garden Party at Wadham College, Oxford, on the occasion of the celebration of the Tercentenary of the foundation of the Royal Society, July 1960. © *Oxford Mail.*

Meade: You have mentioned several people and I think what I will do first of all is to ask them if they want to comment. Can you make your comments and any rebuttals very short and snappy, because we have got quite a lot to get through. John Hampton, would you like to say anything about your work, particularly with Tony Mitchell, whose name quite rightly has been mentioned several times.

Professor John Hampton: I joined Tony in 1964, and by then he had been in platelets quite a long time already.[52] In the nature of things in those days, Sir George Pickering [see Figure 10] and his department in Oxford, was interested in a lot of different topics. He had somebody working on body temperature, somebody working on endothelial cells, and he was doing a lot on blood pressure, and different things of that sort. Now these were little groups of two or three people and I just turned up on the Monday morning, my first day, and Pickering looked at me and said, 'John, oh yes, I think you had better join

[52] Mitchell (1959).

Tony'. And so I became a 'plateleteer', and joined Mike Harrison, who had been there a year longer.

Tony, who was so much at the beginning of platelets, had been involved in two things: one was aggregation, which he had started, and Gustav might be able to put the dates on this. Tony had started doing aggregation by holding platelet-rich plasma up to the light and shaking tubes to see when they went clear. When you could see through the tubes of platelet-rich plasma, the platelets had aggregated. This was a much better technique than Gustav's because the plasma either had aggregated or it hadn't. There was no argument about time course or anything of that sort. He got from there into aggregation *in vivo* and then to his second technique. John Honour had started a technique with an anaesthetized rabbit, where we took a piece of bone from the skull and looked at the blood vessels on the surface of the brain. He pinched an artery with a pair of microtweezers and you could see platelet clumps form and these platelet clumps embolized downstream in the way we now know applies to acute coronary syndromes. One of the things that was of great interest at that time was how these two techniques related to each other, because it became fairly clear that although they had a lot of parallels, there were a lot of differences. Mike should talk about the *Persantin*® story, because there was a great debate as to why *Persantin*® inhibits platelets in the rabbit and did not work in aggregation.[53]

I was given the job of a new technique which was measuring platelet electrophoresis. This was Tony's idea: if two charged cells stuck together then something must happen to their charge when they did so. He had found some weird machine used for other purposes where you peered down a microscope with a stopwatch and you watched platelets float back and forth under an electric field,[54] and again we tried to correlate that with aggregation and to some extent it did and to some extent it didn't. It was a terrible technique, and it drove you mad. It got dropped for the next 30 years after I had finished with it, until Stan Heptinstall produced a paper from someone in the US who had

---

[53] See Appendix 3, note 255 and Glossary, page 160.

[54] Professor John Hampton wrote: 'Hampton and Mitchell developed a tedious visual method of measuring the rate of movement of platelets in an electric field. They found that low concentrations of agents that caused aggregation in platelet-rich plasma (PRP) increased platelet surface charge (an unexpected finding), but higher concentrations caused a decrease in surface charge, which might allow aggregation to occur.' Note on draft transcript, 7 March 2005.

done the whole thing with a laser gadget which was automated and showed exactly what I had shown with Tony 30 years previously.[55] There was not a mention of us at all in their paper. And it was Stanley [Peart], who gave this paper to me to review with a wicked chuckle, and I said, 'This is old hat'. We got a charming letter back from the bloke saying he hadn't checked the literature that far back. I think Mike Harrison could probably say more about *Persantin*®.

Professor Michael Harrison: First, I should say that John's machine was able to tell me when I was about to get flu. The electrophoretic mobility of my platelets changed when I was going to go down with flu, so this technique should not have been dropped. The interest in dipyridamole was of course because Gus had just shown that adenosine and 2-chloro-adenosine were inhibitory and dipyridamole was supposed to be an adenosine–diaminase inhibitor. Tony Mitchell argued that this should increase the effect of endogenous adenosine and would be inhibitory, and we struggled to show a small effect in the *in vitro* aggregometer but were not impressed by it. As John said, when it was used in the context of the *in vivo* model (the injured cortical vessels in the rabbit), it was inhibitory, and this spawned the idea of its clinical use. But these discrepancies between what works in the test tube and what works in an *in vivo* model, and then what actually works in man, continue to be fascinating I think.

Dr Stewart Sage: I suppose I was lucky to be involved in the calcium story quite early on. Measuring calcium in platelets is obviously difficult because of their size [see Figures 1 and 2]. A lot of the earlier techniques precluded their use in platelets, and although there are a few reports of using aequorin in platelets,[56] I suppose the first advance came with the invention of fluorescent calcium indicators that were developed by Roger Tsien.[57] The important thing about these is that they can be loaded into the cell non-disruptively. Roger was working with Tim Rink in the Physiology Laboratory at Cambridge when he developed his first indicator quin-2 and although the first paper I think was actually using lymphocytes, the second paper used human platelets and they tended to use platelets as the favoured cell thereafter.[58]

---

[55] Hampton and Mitchell (1966); Jy *et al.* (1995).

[56] See, for example, Johnson *et al.* (1985).

[57] Tsien (1980).

[58] Rink and Tsien (1982) [human platelets]; Tsien *et al.* (1982) [mouse and pig lymphocytes]; Pozzan *et al.* (1982) [mouse].

I joined Tim's lab as a PhD student, two years after that first calcium paper using platelets in 1981. I was quite lucky to be involved at a very fast-moving time. Roger started developing a lot of much better indicators and I think I am probably one of the first people to have used fura-2, perhaps the most commonly used of the indicators, just because a sample was sent to Tim by Roger Tsien. As fura-2 is much better than quin-2 (you can load much lower concentrations and still get a useful signal) I started to get rather more valuable data. I suppose one of the small contributions that I made was fairly early in the PhD. Tim was sent a contraption by High-Tech Scientific, a company that had been supplying stop-flow apparatus to biochemists and chemists for many years. And Tim said, 'Why don't you play around with this and see if you can use it with whole cells?' Platelets are ideal to be fired through a stop-flow machine without falling apart, which many larger cells clearly do, as has subsequently been discovered. We started to get some information on the kinetics of early calcium changes when platelets were stimulated, which started to shed light on possible underlying mechanisms, and perhaps one of the most important things that grew out of that work was the discovery of what we at the time thought was a very rapid response to ADP, but it was subsequently appreciated through the work of Martyn Mahaut-Smith, who's sitting next to me, it is actually attributable to contaminating ATP. That led on to work with Martyn when he came to Cambridge and carried out the first patch-clamp experiments on stimulated platelets, which is another very important advance, and still a technique that is not often widely used, and I am sure he would like to say something about that. That is how I came into the field and how the calcium story started. Obviously, the use of these calcium indicators has since shed a lot of very useful light on the signalling pathways that are involved in platelet activation.

Dr Martyn Mahaut-Smith: I joined the Department of Physiology in about 1988, actually at the invitation of Tim Rink, who phoned me when I was doing a postdoc in Canada. I had had a very sleepless night after a patching experiment until about 2 o'clock in the morning, when Tim woke me up and said, 'Would you like to come to work in Cambridge on a really exciting project, to work in collaboration with Stewart Sage who is doing this wonderful work using calcium indicators in platelets? It would be a real challenge, that is to try to achieve the first electrophysiological recordings in platelets.' As it turned out, a worker in Japan had just obtained recordings of platelets using the patch-clamp technique, which were published in the

Journal of Physiology.[59] We followed very shortly thereafter with work done in collaboration with Stewart, showing again what we thought were ADP-activated ion channels.[60] These probably represent one of the first events that occur following vascular damage because the kinetics of activation, as Stewart had shown, were within about 10 milliseconds or so and we followed that with patch-clamp recordings showing that this was due to the opening of an ionotropic cation-permeable channel, letting calcium and sodium in. To date we don't really know the role of sodium. Those were really challenging times, just because of the technique, but we did manage to get what we believe were classical recordings. It wasn't until about 2000 that we realized that it was ATP contamination within the ADP that was responsible for activation of the ion channels.[61] Thus these P2X receptors, known now to be $P2X_1$ receptors, are not activated by ADP, but by ATP. I think we still don't understand the relative role of ATP in the activation of platelets. It was Professor Born who showed that ATP goes up quite considerably following vascular damage.[62] I think it is a really exciting area and is still being carried forward now that we know there are three platelet P2 receptors. Following on from the topic of this meeting about why particular experiments were done, and how they advanced knowledge of platelets and platelet ion channels, we now do our electrophysiological recordings on megakarocytes. They are a 1000 times the capacitance of a platelet, and we feel that in many respects they represent giant, nucleated platelets.[63] So because of the relative ease of those patch-clamp experiments on the megakaroctye, I believe that there are exciting times ahead, particularly for studies of platelet ion channels.

Meade: Colin Prentice, you were mentioned by Stan Heptinstall, do you want to add anything at this stage?

Professor Colin Prentice: My experience with platelet involvement started with Stuart Douglas and George McNicol in Glasgow,[64] which was another centre of enthusiasts working away, and certainly Born and Cross's

---

[59] Maruyama (1987).

[60] Mahaut-Smith *et al.* (1990).

[61] Mahaut-Smith *et al.* (2000).

[62] Born and Kratzer (1984).

[63] Mahaut-Smith *et al.* (2003).

[64] Prentice *et al.* (1966). See also, for example, McNicol and Douglas (1964).

aggregometry was a very powerful tool at this early stage. Another person who made a big impact in the 1960s was Hellem with his glass-bead columns.[65] I think we must acknowledge one or two of the pioneers, and he really developed the very exciting work that when you ran the blood through the glass-bead columns there was platelet disappearance, because the platelets aggregated due to substances, later found to be ADP, which were released from the red cells. This was one of the foundation clues that led to the discovery that ADP aggregated platelets. Another person on the continent was Bounameaux,[66] who I think was probably the first to show that an extract of macerated arterial vessel was a powerful and permanent aggregator of platelets. Now I may be wrong, he may not have used the collagenase, but shortly after that he discovered that this arterial component was collagen. I think it was these two biological experiments that led to the concept that collagen was a powerful platelet aggregator. Thus, you have the two components for platelet aggregation, the ADP short reversible aggregation, and the collagen, which irreversibly aggregates platelets after a latent period of half a minute or so. This we now know is due to the release of thromboxanes mediated by the prostaglandin cycle, which leads to the slower irreversibile platelet aggregation. I think these individuals were important at the stage when we were working up in Glasgow.

Our group in Glasgow went on to look at another platelet adhesive factor, the factor VIII-related antigen, the von Willebrand factor, and that was another exciting story which developed in the 1970s.[67] It took quite a long time to work out the difference between haemophiliacs and von Willebrand disease patients, which was a mystery in the 1970s. Inga Marie Nilsson showed in 1957 that if you infused normal serum into von Willebrand disease patients – an experiment that I don't think is very ethical nowadays – that it shortened their bleeding time and this was due to the von Willebrand factor which was being injected into the von Willebrand disease patients.[68] It was later discovered that von Willebrand factor enables platelet adhesion to take place in normal people. Lack of von Willebrand factor causes defective platelet

[65] Hellem (1960).

[66] Bounameaux and Roskam (1959).

[67] See Tansey and Christie (1999): 72–4, 81, with photographs of early apparatus used in the preparation of animal antihaemophilic globulin in 1955 on pages 48–51.

[68] Nilsson *et al.* (1957). See also Nilsson (1994).

adhesion and a prolonged bleeding time in affected patients. So I think in addition to the ADP–collagen story, others would like to take up the von Willebrand factor and fibrinogen as components of platelet aggregation and adhesion, and the glycoprotein one as well.

Meade: May I just pause at this moment to say that although this is a UK audience, we did ask some people from overseas, but they couldn't come. Of course, a great deal of the work that we are concerned with has taken part in this country, but I think we shouldn't forget that many investigators elsewhere have made important contributions.[69]

Professor Peter Elwood: Before we leave the UK, may I mention John O'Brien? In the year that Gus Born published his landmark paper on platelet aggregation in 1962, in that same year John O'Brien totally independently published a paper on platelet aggregation.[70] So perhaps what Gus very graciously said, that it didn't require a great intellectual leap to develop the technique, is true. But John O'Brien was an enormous encourager and a tremendous help to many in their work on platelets and he remained active working on platelets and on platelet technology up into his 80s.[71] Unfortunately, he died earlier this year,[72] but he brought out a method of shear-stress activation of platelets that we incorporated into one of our epidemiological studies.[73] Sadly, it did not predict MI [myocardial infarction], but neither does the Born method of platelet aggregation.

Born: I have to come back on that. I am sorry that John O'Brien may have convinced himself that he invented the optical aggregometer, but the fact of the matter is that it had been demonstrated to him by myself in my department some time before he published it without acknowledgement to me. This is confirmed by a letter from Sir John Vane who was present at the same time as my senior lecturer.[74]

Professor Donald Chambers: My work on platelets from 1963 to 1969 began in a fortuitous way. I had a laboratory at the Massachusetts General Hospital,

---

[69] For Harvey Weiss's personal recollections of platelet work in North America, see Weiss (2003).

[70] O'Brien (1962).

[71] Sharp *et al.* (1990).

[72] For further details of his work, see Ness *et al.* (2002), 74–5, 128.

[73] Beswick *et al.* (1994).

[74] See note 12.

Boston, just down the hall from Edwin Salzman. At the time I was working on proteases and the mechanisms of acute pancreatitis. One morning Ed came to see me and said, 'I need your advice. Given the fact that thrombin relates to platelet aggregation, what do you think would happen if you added proteolytic synthetic substrate, benzoyl-L-arginine methyl ester synthetic substrate, to platelet-rich plasma?' I responded, 'My bet is that it would inhibit platelet aggregation, because it would act as a competitive substrate to thrombin'. Ed did the experiment and returned two days later. 'You were right,' he said. That started a six-year collaboration that subsequently moved to the Beth Israel Hospital, Boston [now Beth Israel Deaconess Medical Center], examining the mechanisms of platelet aggregation.[75] We asked such questions as: what are the dynamics of platelet aggregation?; how does ADP aggregate platelets?; what is the nucleotide metabolism of platelets? At times, we incubated platelets with ^{14}C-labelled ADP and ^{32}P-ADP, lysed them, and found that ^{14}C-ADP was taken up by platelets, probably in the form of adenosine, but ^{32}P-ADP was not. Additionally, much of the ADP released by platelets was nonradioactive, suggesting nucleotide compartmentalization.[76] We ended our close scientific collaboration with a hypothesis about the energy state of platelets and the role of platelet cell surface ecto-ATPases (published in *Nature*): we presented the argument that the non-sticky state of the platelet represented its active state and when platelets died, they entered a less active state and aggregated.[77] That hypothesis caused a lot of discussion, which I think is a hallmark of science.

Another thing we were into early was the role of cyclic AMP (cAMP) in platelet metabolism and function. Ed Salzman was an early pioneer in investigating that cAMP was protective against platelet aggregation, which I think was a breakthrough and preceded the mechanistic understanding of how prostacyclines work.[78] By that time I had left Boston, but continued to explore the role of cAMP in biological systems at Columbia University, New York, where we studied cAMP in the regulation of the *E. coli* gene cluster, the *lac* operon, leading to the isolation of a cAMP DNA-binding protein, which was the first positive gene regulatory protein to be discovered and isolated. Since then I have gone on to investigate interactions between catecholamines and

---

[75] Salzman and Chambers (1964).

[76] See note 9.

[77] Salzman *et al.* (1966).

[78] See, for example, Salzman (1972, 1976).

cAMP in regulating immune function, and mediating interactions between the nervous system and the immune system.

Something we need to remember about platelet research in the US in the 1960s is that it was performed by a comparatively small group: Ted Spaet, Aaron Marcus, Marjorie Zucker and Ralph Nachman were the leading researchers, and we all knew one another.[79] Although there was individual competition, it was much less than that which I think now characterizes science; possibly because money flowed from the National Institutes of Health (NIH) in the 1960s, and those halcyon days are over.

Meade: Thank you very much. My apologies for assuming that this was an all-Brit[ish] audience. I am very glad that you made that contribution. Michael Oliver do you want to say something?

Professor Michael Oliver: My contribution, Tom, really is historical. In 1954, working in Edinburgh, we had pretty well defined the lipoprotein profile in normal people and in coronary patients. I was working with George Boyd in considerable isolation and was concerned, maybe because we were in Scotland, that nobody else seemed to be the least bit interested in atherosclerosis. So I took myself off to meet John French in Oxford. This was 1958. The Great Western Railway was late by 20 minutes, and John met me at the station in a terrible flap, as he had bicycled down from the Dunn School of Pathology. He said, 'Could you afford a taxi? Prof has got a lecture at five past 1 o'clock and he's waiting for you.' Now, I hadn't done my homework, I didn't know who Prof was. When I went up the stairs, at the double, there was this steely grey-haired man whom I later recognized as Howard Florey. He said, 'If you want to try to form an atherosclerosis group go ahead, but it won't work, because there aren't more than nine people in the country who are the least bit interested in the subject, and you have got three of them here, you, French and me.' He then produced a bottle of white wine out of his desk with three glasses, one for himself before the lecture, and one for each of us, and poured half the bottle into the glasses. He told me to go away and find 20 people, and he told French to find £250 a year. He told us to come back in three months, which we duly did. This time French and I met, and prepared our brief before meeting the Nobel Prize winner. We thought we had better get it right. I found 18 people, and French had got £250 for three years from ICI – a lot of money

[79] For a photograph of some of those mentioned, see Weiss (2003): 1874. A note on his US platelet research experiences by Professor Donald Chambers has been deposited in the Wellcome Library, London, along with the notes and records of this meeting.

in those days. We went through the list and Florey removed three people, whom I shall not name, from the list. He asked about Helen Payling-Wright, Gwyn MacFarlane and Rosemary Biggs. 'Why hadn't I included them?' So these three replaced the three Florey didn't like, or who were rivals or whatever, and off we set with the Atherosclerosis Discussion Group, now the British Atherosclerosis Society.[80] To initiate it, Florey again produced a half bottle of white wine and three glasses. Now, to this day I do not know whether that was the same bottle of white wine or not.

Meade: Stan Peart, you came across platelets in a slightly different context, I think, earlier on perhaps than we have so far heard. Would you like to say something about that?

Professor Sir Stanley Peart: I regard platelets as a damn nuisance, actually. The reason for my saying so is that I was in J H Gaddum's department in Edinburgh in 1946 and I was struggling to demonstrate the amines coming off the sympathetic nerve endings when they were stimulated. I can remember at that time it was uncertain whether it was adrenaline or noradrenaline. And what I discovered – because I was using smooth muscle of different sorts, including isolated arteries to demonstrate what the substances were – that plasma unfortunately constricted blood vessels and contracted smooth muscle rather well, except I didn't know what the substances were and in 1946, it wasn't very clear what they were. Spinning the blood very hard to get rid of the platelets did not remove this effect, and, of course, that led me back into history: first to Otto Loewi, 1921, who is worth mentioning, because he coined the phrases *acceleranstöf* and *vagusstöf* in relation to quickening and slowing the heart rate on sympathetic or vagal stimulation. That led me back to Ernest Starling and the big efforts made to do heart–lung perfusion, which they discovered they could not easily do. And even if they filtered the plasma to get rid of what they

---

[80] Professor Michael Oliver wrote: 'Florey was the first chairman of the Atherosclerosis Discussion Group and George Pickering the second. The first meeting was held in MRC head office in Queen Anne's Gate, London. There was a debate on the function of platelets and the relevance of platelet adhesiveness to atherosclerosis and coronary disease. Papers were presented by Tony Mitchell, John O'Brien and Helen Payling Wright. This was, possibly, the first serious discussion of the subject, arising from Gustav Born's seminal report. I was the secretary of the Group and my recollection is that Lawson McDonald (London), Brian Bronte-Stewart (Glasgow), Gerry Shaper (London) and Elspeth Smith (Aberdeen) also participated. Thereafter the Group met twice each year – at Magdalen College, Oxford, in the spring and Jesus College, Cambridge, in the autumn. There were many papers and discussions on the relations among platelets, thrombosis and atherosclerosis.' Note on draft transcript, 5 May 2004. For further details see: www.britathsoc.ac.uk/ (visited 3 February 2005).

thought were small aggregates, it still contracted the heart–lung preparation in different ways and damaged the heart in various ways. Perfused blood contained *frühgift*, which dilated blood vessels and *spätgift*, which contracted them.[81]

From my point of view, because of these substances I could not assay what turned out to be noradrenaline in the plasma after the sympathetic nerves had been stimulated. I then discovered by chance, not with any hypothesis-driven ideas, that dihydro-ergotamine would block the *spätgift*. So I used dihydro-ergotamine and was able to assay on the smooth muscle of blood vessels, the noradrenaline and maybe small traces of adrenalin present when you stimulated the sympathetic nerves. Soon afterwards it was discovered that platelets released 5-hydroxytryptamine, known as serotonin or *spätgift*, and it was this substance that dihydro-ergotamine was blocking.

Professor Rod Flower: I would like to comment on Gus Born's technique, because I think that while it obviously had an enormous utility for the study of events in haemostasis, it has another great utility as well: it was probably the first technique that was available whereby people could easily investigate the pharmacology of a single human cell type and as a teaching tool it has been absolutely fantastic. You can teach many basic pharmacological principles, such as agonism, antagonism, physiological antagonism and so on, with this very simple technique, using human cells and since there is only one cell type present there is no confusion about the results. It has been a really remarkable technique for all sorts of reasons other than the one for which you invented it, Gus.

Meade: I think we will move on now, and I will say a few words about the relationship of platelets to thrombotic disorders.

There's obviously been no doubt for a long time about the involvement of platelets in thrombosis, and so that does naturally raise the question of whether there might be some tests that would pick out people who are at risk of thrombosis and clinical coronary disease, because of the instability or sensitivity – or whatever the right word would be – of their platelets. In about 1980 we went to see Gustav to introduce platelet aggregometry into the Northwick Park Heart Study using his method.[82] Now I have to say that right

---

[81] Loewi (1953). For the background to Loewi's work, see his Nobel lecture at http://nobelprize.org/medicine/laureates/1936/loewi-lecture.html (visited 14 March 2005).

[82] The Northwick Park Heart Study recruited its population of 1510 white men aged 40–64 years between 1972 and 1978 and the study was supported in part by the British Heart Foundation. See Meade *et al.* (1980, 1986).

from the start Gustav said he didn't think his method had got anything to do with thrombosis. But I was pretty sure that I had read a paper somewhere that he had written saying that it did.[83] We decided to introduce his methods. I think probably our data on this are the most comprehensive. We measured aggregation to platelets using both adrenaline and ADP in plasma that had been standardized for its platelet count, and we measured the maximum response and the ED_{50} [effective $dose_{50}$ is the amount of material required to produce a specified effect in 50 per cent of the population being studied]. From an epidemiological point of view, the first thing is to see whether these measures are related to other well-known risk factors for coronary disease. What turned out was that in some respects they were. For example, aggregability seemed to increase with age and to be less in people according to the amount of alcohol they took, and that seemed to make a certain amount of sense. On the other hand, there were some very unexpected findings, of which the most striking without any doubt at all was that nonsmokers had more aggregable platelets than smokers. I don't know what the explanation for that would be. Incidentally, I think I should mention at this point that of course the platelet system is only part of the haemostatic system as a whole, and other aspects have already been mentioned. The effect that thrombin has on platelet aggregability may be very important and also the effect that the fibrinogen level may have.

The next stage for the epidemiologist is to look at people who have already had a heart attack and to compare them with people who haven't, because that's something you can do relatively easily. The problem about that approach is that of course you can't include people who have died of coronary episodes, which certainly are going to be of particular interest. I have always wondered whether we can pinpoint differences between people who survive heart attacks and people who don't, or whether it is just a matter of chance. And then there's always the problem in these cross-sectional studies that you can't be sure whether what you find may not have been influenced by the previous event itself, and also by the changes in lifestyle that people have put themselves through or have been advised to take. Peter Elwood and his colleagues in the Caerphilly–Speedwell Study[84] did that and in a minute, Peter, I will ask you to say something about that study.

---

[83] Professor Gustav Born wrote: 'The paper Tom was referring to was my 1962b paper in *Nature*, where I comment on the possible prevention of thrombosis by platelet inhibitors.' Note on draft transcript, 25 February 2005.

[84] See Ness *et al.* (2002) and note 89.

But the most important approach for the epidemiologist, short of randomized-controlled trials, which we will come on to later, is the cohort or prospective study where you characterize people in a number of ways, including their platelet function, before the event, and then see what happens to them later on. That has been approached in two ways: first of all in terms of people who have actually already had an event and who have been followed up for a recurrent event. There are two well-known studies on this: one by Trip and others published in 1990, who found that spontaneous platelet aggregation appeared to be associated with an increased risk of a recurrent event;[85] the other is the work by John Martin, who unfortunately isn't here today, and his colleagues showing that platelet size appeared to be related to a recurrent event.[86] We could have some discussion about what the interpretation of that observation might be. But that leads on to the second approach, of what predicts first events, in other words in people who so far have not had a coronary event. As far as I can see, the first substantial report on this was by a Norwegian group in 1991, who reported that mortality from coronary disease was considerably reduced in those with higher platelet counts and also who had particularly aggregable platelets to ADP.[87]

By 1997 we had been able to follow up the people on whom we had initially carried out Gustav's aggregometry and we found no relationship whatever between the incidence of coronary heart disease (CHD) and either of the aggregating agents, nor within each aggregating agent, the different parameters that we had used, and furthermore, platelet count appeared not to be related to it either. We had also been using the Hellem technique for platelet adhesiveness to glass beads.[88] From an epidemiological point of view [this] is of no value, because it is so variable. If you do it on somebody's sample now, it will give you quite a different answer in a sample than tomorrow morning or evening. Peter Elwood can also tell us about the results in the Caerphilly–Speedwell studies, where they also found no relationship, and I will give him a chance to go into that in just a moment.[89]

---

[85] Trip *et al.* (1990).

[86] Martin *et al.* (1991).

[87] Thaulow *et al.* (1991).

[88] Hellem (1960).

[89] Dr Peter Elwood described the background to the Caerphilly project in an interview with Dr Andy Ness on 28 February 2001. See Appendix 1, page 81. See also Ness *et al.* (2002).

So as far as trying to characterize people who are at risk of coronary events because of anything to do with their platelets, I think we are no further on than we were when we started. There's no question about the involvement of platelets in coronary disease, and that's something that I think we don't need to debate. But I don't think we have any idea really about how to characterize people who may have run into trouble because of something to do with their platelets. That's my view anyway. Now, Peter, I have mentioned you and you mentioned your own study earlier, so would you like to tell us about both the cross-sectional and the prospective findings in that study.

Elwood: Like you, Mr Chairman, we didn't put a lot of weight on the cross-sectional data, that is platelet function in men who had already had a heart attack and I really would prefer not to say anything about that, because I don't remember the results. I think far more important is that in the Caerphilly study we did platelet tests on more than 2000 middle-aged men. We did platelet aggregation in platelet-rich plasma (PRP), and we did platelet aggregation in whole blood using the Flower aggregometer method.[90] We also did platelet aggregation by the shear-stress method, developed by John O'Brien,[91] and we did a very crude bleeding time test, but believed to be a global test of haemostasis, and in particular a measure, however crude, of platelet function. We looked at the reproducibility of these tests, and a lot of other tests, both within the laboratory, and over time within subjects. While reproducibility within subjects over a period of weeks was not as good as other measures, like cholesterol, blood pressure etc., still the coefficient of variation was only about 15 per cent and we felt that with the large numbers we had we should detect any prediction, if there was prediction.[92] We have followed up these men, are still following them up, and we had about 200 new events of MI and over 100 ischaemic strokes. We found that none of these tests – PRP aggregation, whole-blood aggregation, shear-stress aggregation and bleeding time – showed prediction of MI, not even a hint of prediction of MI.[93] We did find a weak prediction of ischaemic stroke, but it was the reverse of what we had expected. The men with the more active platelets, whether judged in aggregation or bleeding time, the more active the platelets, the lower the

---

[90] Cardinal and Flower (1979, 1980).

[91] O'Brien and Salmon (1990).

[92] Elwood *et al.* (1993).

[93] Elwood *et al.* (2001, 2003).

subsequent incidence of ischaemic stroke. I have discussed this with a number of plateletologists, and haematologists, but no-one has come up with any reasonable explanation of those findings. Unlike what you and Gus Born say now, I did expect that platelet aggregation would predict MI. Perhaps that just shows how naive I am, but furthermore, I certainly wouldn't have expected it to predict stroke the wrong way round according to what we thought was a reasonable expectation.

Born: Right at the very beginning I should have put some kind of toxicity warning on the method, 'not good for clinical use'; but you, Tom, and I have often discussed this and I was with you for trying it out. I am glad to know the results; they are not surprising, but I simply wondered whether a ruptured plaque isn't such an overwhelming pathological event that if you think of the real situation, with red cells and everything going round, whatever small changes there may be in platelets would be a rather minor variant in something which is overwhelming in other ways.

Elwood: What about stroke? Can I ask Gus about stroke? Why does platelet aggregation weakly predict stroke the wrong way round?

Meade: Was it a chance finding? What sort of level of significance was there?

Elwood: The significance of some of the tests was below the conventional level, but it was a consistent trend in four approaches to platelet aggregation, in PRP, and whole blood, and shear stress, and the bleeding time.

Meade: I suppose it could have been chance.

Elwood: Anything can be chance, but it's rather strange.

Heptinstall: Some years ago we did quite extensive investigations of post-MI patients and we thought we had identified something rather interesting. We had set ourselves up to measure the platelet-release reaction. We labelled platelets in platelet-rich plasma (PRP) with ^{14}C-serotonin and then looked at how much of the serotonin was released from the platelets when they were stimulated with ADP. We compared the results obtained for healthy controls with those for people studied immediately post-MI, and there was a significant difference between the two. Significantly more release occurred in the MI group than in the control group. There was, however, a huge overlap of individual results within the two groups. About a year later we looked back at the data, at who in the MI group had survived this event and who had not. We saw that there was far greater release reaction in the patients who didn't survive their MI compared with those who did. We tried to pass that technique on to

Tom to use in his Northwick Park study but somehow the technique didn't transfer very well and they didn't take it up.[94] Nevertheless there was a hint of something interesting.

Here is another anecdote. We were asked by our clinical colleagues to look at platelets from a patient who had a very high platelet count and was having some sort of neurological problems, despite the fact that he was taking aspirin. His platelet count was about 1 million platelets per microlitre [the normal platelet count is 150 000–350 000 per microlitre of blood]. At the time one of the platelet parameters that we were able to measure was spontaneous platelet aggregation in whole blood. All we did was to take whole blood, stir it and look at the disappearance of platelets. It seemed to me that there was no point in looking at his platelets while he was taking aspirin, because the aspirin might have interfered with the measurements we were to perform and consequently his aspirin was withdrawn. We then took a blood sample and what we found was staggering. As soon as we stirred the blood, all the platelets aggregated together. There was no need to add an agonist, they just aggregated together spontaneously. It was the biggest spontaneous platelet aggregation we had ever seen, and far greater than for other people in the same age range. Clearly the man's platelets were very hyperactive. At the same time we looked at the ability of prostacyclin and prostaglandin D_2 to inhibit platelet aggregation, and basically we couldn't inhibit the aggregation using these agents. Please bear in mind that all of this was before aspirin was clearly established as an antithrombotic agent. About a week following our determinations, the patient had a stroke and died.

Meade: Because you had taken him off aspirin?

Heptinstall: Well, maybe. What I would say is that I would never ask for anybody to be taken off aspirin again. But let me also say again, all this happened before the time that we were convinced of the therapeutic value of aspirin. I firmly believe that this was a very atypical situation where someone had a very high platelet count, the platelets seemed to be unresponsive to natural inhibitors of platelet aggregation, and were demonstrably hyperactive. I believe that the platelet hyperaggregability contributed to the stroke.

Meade: That's a bit like the Trip study, isn't it?

---

[94] See note 82.

Heptinstall: The Trip people showed spontaneous platelet aggregation in platelet-rich plasmas.[95] I have to say I don't understand spontaneous aggregation in platelet-rich plasma. I don't know what's causing it. I do understand it in whole blood to a certain extent, in that it's almost impossible to do anything with whole blood without damaging red cells. The red cells release not only ADP, but also huge amounts of ATP, both of which can cause platelet aggregation. You may be interested to hear that we have just published a paper showing for the first time that ATP added to whole blood causes extensive platelet aggregation, and it does so by virtue of the white cells and ecto-ATPases which are able to convert the ATP into ADP and bring about the aggregation response.[96]

Oliver: Concerning stroke: let's not lose track of the fact that such a clinical diagnosis covers at least three major entities and that about less than half of so-called clinical strokes are thrombotics – haemorrhagic stroke, and stroke resulting from degenerative cerebral changes with advancing age account for many. The person who's shown this most clearly is Jack Strong, with his enormous survey in the US, with over 20 000 autopsies.[97] To wonder why one cannot see such and such a change in platelets in relationship to stroke, I think, is naive, because the causes of stroke are multiple and not all thrombotic. The underlying pathology is the key.

Professor Salvador Moncada: I just wanted to make a comment that follows on from what you have just said, Michael. It is impossible to predict the outcome when you are looking at only one of the factors involved in thrombosis. There are at least three different components that play a role in the final common event, which is a stroke or MI. The behaviour of platelets alone would not be an adequate predictor. On the other hand, we are talking about two things: one is the final event (a thrombotic one) and the other is the role that platelets play in the development of the disease. The interplay of the two factors might be different in the two processes and may again differ between individuals in a population. In the last 25 years we have learnt how important the vessel wall is – it is not just a surface where platelets stick.

---

95 Trip *et al.* (1990).

96 Stafford *et al.* (2003).

97 McGill *et al.* (2000).

So the platelet aggregometry *in vitro* is a great technique that has been immensely useful in understanding platelet behaviour. However, what platelets do *in vivo* is what matters. Gus probably never thought that aggregometry alone would be sufficient.[98]

Meade: I think it's worth pointing out that the coagulation system actually has been much more rewarding in trying to explain the thrombotic aspects of coronary heart disease.

Dr Peter Hunter: I would like to comment on how treatments are actually discovered as opposed to the published accounts, for example, platelet aggregation in diabetes, especially in relation to retinopathy. Dr Henry Heath at the University College Hospital Medical School, London, from 1968 to 1970 worked on diabetes, and the importance of his research turned out to lie primarily in the experimental design rather than the aggregation results. He compared 25 diabetics with rapidly deteriorating haemorrhagic retinopathy with 25 diabetics of more than 15 years' duration with no or minimal diabetic retinopathy. They were compared for 80 variables and one of these variables – cutaneous capillary resistance (the capacity of the capillary wall to resist rupture by increased pressure in the lumen, or reduced pressure, a vacuum, outside the vessel, or both) – turned out to be highly significant.[99] The patients who were deteriorating had very low capillary resistance and their capillaries would bleed very fast. The immune diabetics not only had very high capillary resistance, but were within the range of the nondiabetic population.

Meade: I am not sure how much progress in terms of actually predicting coronary events we have made on this front. I think the answer is not much. Now we will move on to: the platelet release reaction; aspirin in relation to that; and also some comments about inflammation. I will ask Duncan Thomas first of all to comment.

Dr Duncan Thomas: I have been asked to concentrate on the start of the story of aspirin and platelets, mainly because the prime movers are dead or can't be with us today. The key observations were made over a short period of time, a relatively few months in the mid-1960s.

---

[98] See quantitative methods for measuring haemostatic/thrombotic platelet aggregation *in vivo* in Born *et al.* (1964); Born and Philip (1965); Begent and Born (1970); Richardson *et al.* (1976); Zawilska *et al.* (1982); Kortenhaus *et al.* (1982); Begent *et al.* (1983).

[99] Heath *et al.* (1971).

For me, the story started in the summer of 1966, when I had just joined Gus Born and worked in his lab for a year on sabbatical. A paper appeared in *Nature* from D C Macmillan, who was working with Michael Oliver in Edinburgh, and he was the first to show clearly the second phase of platelet aggregation.[100] He showed that there was a primary phase resulting from the added agonist and then release of the endogenous nucleotides and other components leading to the second phase of aggregation. We were all a bit miffed at this, because many of us had seen the phenomenon, as 'through a glass darkly', but hadn't really appreciated the significance. But Macmillan had, and this observation became an essential part of the story of aspirin and platelets. Aggregometry may not be very good at predicting MI, but it works very well in analysing how aspirin works.

The next part of the story that I remember was the Miemo meeting[101] in Italy in September 1967, which some people here will recall.[102] The only person who talked about aspirin, platelets and thrombosis was Breddin from Frankfurt,[103] who had spotted a letter in the *Lancet* in the spring of 1967 by C D W Morris, who said that he had given aspirin to 35 subjects and shown that it had dramatically impaired aggregation, using the Born aggregometer.[104] To the best of my knowledge, that's the first published evidence linking aspirin and impaired platelet aggregation. Breddin had taken it to the stage where he was routinely giving his patients 1g or 2g of aspirin every day for thrombotic

---

[100] Macmillan (1966).

[101] Professor Donald Chambers wrote: 'Another memorable but less traumatic meeting [see note 162] occurred in 1967 at Castel Miemo, Miemo, an Italian hamlet, near Pisa. This conference had as an objective the assembly of all the information then available concerning the role of platelets in haemostasis, to define knowledge gaps so as to provide a framework for further research [Haanen and Jürgens (eds) (1968)]. About 50 scientists representing at least ten countries, met at the Pisa airport and were driven by coach to the baronial estate of a scion of the Italian pharmaceutical industry, where for three days we were treated to three-course breakfasts, four-course luncheons, and six-course banquet dinners. The active meetings were punctuated by frequent breaks for pastry, juice, coffee and tea, and the accommodation included vast rooms, marble bathrooms and luxuries that few of us were accustomed to. The scientific meetings were organized in a discussion format such that everyone had a preprint of the paper under discussion. Even the slide projectionist, a graduate student of Professor Born, asked questions. All in all, it was a meeting that the attendees still talk about and remember fondly.' E-mail to Mrs Lois Reynolds, 7 April 2005.

[102] Breddin (1967).

[103] See also note 179.

[104] Morris (1967). See also Morris and Miller (1966).

disorders, although at no time did he claim that he was doing a clinical trial. But at this meeting in September 1967 nobody else talked about aspirin and platelets. However, that very month, Harvey Weiss and Lou Aledort in New York published a paper in the *Lancet* which showed that in ten subjects (six of them were physicians, so it was clearly a lab study) given 1.3g of aspirin a day for a couple of days, aggregation induced by connective tissue was impaired.[105] This was not the case when they used ADP, interestingly, although they missed that, and they also missed the second phase of aggregation. But they did conclusively show that aggregation by collagen was impaired by aspirin, and this is, I think, generally regarded as the first decent paper showing that aspirin impaired platelet aggregation.

Now Weiss and Aledort were very restrained. The only thing they said in the discussion, the final sentence, was: 'the results suggest that these agents may have antithrombotic properties'. That was the only comment they allowed themselves at the time. Later, they went on to demonstrate the second phase of aggregation, but they did not comment on it in that early paper. A few months later in January 1968, John O'Brien wrote a letter to the *Lancet* in which he showed that the secondary wave of aggregation produced by adrenalin is inhibited by aspirin.[106] And then hot on his heels in March 1968, an important paper was published by Marjorie Zucker in New York.[107] She gave ten subjects 1.3g of aspirin and showed that secondary aggregation, serotonin release and platelet factor 3 (PF3) activation induced by ADP were abolished by aspirin. She concluded that aspirin should be added to the list of drugs that prevent platelet aggregation induced by ADP. Being a PhD [not an MD] she didn't get into the clinical aspects, but she showed how aspirin works by impairing the release reaction. Quite independently, Fraser Mustard's group at McMaster University in Canada was looking at the same problem from an experimental point of view. They showed that aspirin given to their animals impaired thrombosis in extracorporeal shunts.[108]

The next part of the story is in April 1968 when John O'Brien confirmed that the second wave of aggregation after ADP was abolished by aspirin, and showed there was also a poor response to collagen after aspirin. And he

---

[105] Weiss and Aledort (1967).

[106] O'Brien (1968a).

[107] Zucker and Peterson (1968).

[108] Mustard *et al.* (1967); Evans *et al.* (1968). For a more recent review, see Mustard and Packham (1977).

reported that the effect was produced by a small dose of 150mg. Everybody before O'Brien had been giving gram amounts, but he showed that it only needed 150mg to have an effect, and to the best of my knowledge he was the first to show this. His last couple of sentences in that paper are worth repeating because they are quite prophetic:

> the abnormalities following aspirin ingestion which I have described are quite sufficient to justify a therapeutic trial of aspirin in individuals at risk of thrombosis. Aspirin is relatively safe, and is used probably more than any other drug and nobody knows whether it decreases thrombosis or not.[109]

Clearly the ground had been set up for Peter Elwood's trial, which we will hear about later. I think one should acknowledge that O'Brien was the first to suggest that somebody should do a clinical trial to see if these observations, that everybody by now had seen in the lab, had clinical relevance. It's very interesting how quickly all these events happened, in a matter of a few months in 1967/8.

The next phase in the story is 1970/1, which I am sure Rod Flower will tell us about, where the mechanism of action of aspirin was worked out by John Vane, Bryan Smith and Jim Willis.

Meade: Thank you very much, Duncan. We mustn't overlook the inflammatory aspect of coronary disease and the effect of aspirin on inflammation, and so I hope Clive Page will spend just a few minutes talking about that.

Professor Clive Page: I am not actually going to talk at all about coronary disease. I came into the platelet field really working at what is now the National Heart and Lung Institute, [then called] the Cardiothoracic Institute at the Brompton Hospital. I was working with Dr John Morley, who at the time was the Director (1979/80–84) of the Asthma Research Council's clinical pharmacology unit. He had been approached by Alan White and Keith Butler of what was then Ciba-Geigy Pharmaceuticals in Horsham [Ciba Laboratories, Horsham, later the Ciba-Geigy Pharmaceuticals Division and now Novartis], to really try and find a way of automating *in vivo* what Gus had done *in vitro.* We established a method to use the lung as a filter to look at the accumulation of platelet aggregates in the pulmonary vascular bed by monitoring platelets

---

109 O'Brien (1968b): 783.

radio-labelled with indium.[110] This was my thesis work and until that point at Ciba-Geigy they were actually injecting animals with ADP or some other thrombotic stimulus and at intervals of one minute, two minutes, three minutes, four minutes, they were sacrificing animals, taking out lungs, and actually counting the aggregates histologically, which is a very tedious process requiring a lot of animals. We were, in effect, asked to try to see if we could simplify this and study platelet aggregation *in vivo* in real time, as Salvador said, with all the other components in place. And I think we were successful in doing that, and we developed what, in effect, became a noninvasive way of looking at platelet function *in vivo*. But because we were a lung group we were interested in also measuring lung function in these animals, and we found that with certain stimuli, particularly platelet-activating factor (PAF), we not only got embolization of platelets that was reversible within the pulmonary vascular bed, but we were getting changes in lung mechanics.

Going back to 1954 and the work of Professor John Widdicombe, who first described airway reflexes in response to pulmonary embolism, we had just assumed that it would be physical obstruction of the pulmonary vasculature that triggered this.[111] It turned out to be far from that and we actually went on to show, as Boris Vargaftig's group did in the Pasteur Institute in Paris, that platelets could, in response to PAF, be found extravascularly alongside airway smooth muscle tissue with inflammatory cells, and at the time we really didn't understand this observation. However, it was clear that there wasn't a full-blown thrombosis with coagulation, these were platelets behaving as primitive leukocytes, and of course many years earlier others had suggested that in certain lower organisms, platelets can behave as primitive leukocytes.[112]

We went on from there to really investigate this further, and I think it's very clear from the work that we performed with Jim Metzger's group in the US in about 1990, if my memory serves me correctly.[113] When we made allergic animals thrombocytopaenic by removing more than 95 per cent of their circulating platelets, we saw absolutely no recruitment of leukocytes into lung tissue in response to an allergen stimulus, and we came to the conclusion at the time that platelets were not just there as innocent bystanders, but were actively participating in some way in recruiting leukocytes into tissue.

---

[110] Page *et al.* (1982). 111-Indium-labelled homologous platelets were used. See also Morley (1977).

[111] Widdicombe (1954).

[112] Gordon and Milner (1976).

[113] Coyle *et al.* (1990).

Over the last ten years my own group has provided further evidence supporting this whole idea that platelets are inflammatory cells. We have recently reported that in patients with clinical asthma, if you take blood samples from such patients undergoing an asthma attack, you will find platelets coating leukocytes. You don't see really thrombocytopaenia and aggregation, you see platelets coating leukocytes. If we add platelets to leukocytes in a culture, we get greater leukocyte adhesion to vascular endothelium as the platelet levels in normal circulating blood.[114] From our pharmacological studies, we know this is completely insensitive to aspirin, so there's a novel mechanism underlying this behaviour of platelets in terms of signaling, in comparison with all of the work that has been discussed prior to this in the context of thrombosis.

I think it reflects a completely different function that platelets have in the body, in that they are actually part of the defence mechanism and in regulating leukocyte recruitment. Of course if you look at the literature, there are a lot of parallels with metastasis of tumour cells, where in animal models, if you make animals thromocytopaenic, the tumour doesn't metastasize to the same extent, particularly if you look at lung tumours.[115] I think tumour cells often use similar mechanisms described in leukocytes, such as integrin-type mechanisms to get out into tissue.[116]

This is a completely different aspect of platelet biology which we stumbled upon totally by accident, because we happened to be measuring the lung or using the lung as an organ for the read-out of the particular phenomenon we were interested in.

Meade: Good, thank you very much. Has anybody got any views about coronary disease and aspirin dose, since this is a question that is often asked?

Moncada: If you are talking about 75mg or 150mg of aspirin a day you are not going to affect the inflammatory process to any significant degree. The effects you see with these doses are more related to platelets, rather than to inflammation.

---

[114] Pitchford *et al.* (2003, 2004).

[115] Jamieson and Scipio (eds) (1982).

[116] Vlodavsky and Friedmann (2001).

Elwood: I think it was Ridker who looked at the physicians' aspirin study in the US.[117] There they used alternate doses of 100mg of aspirin and he showed a significant effect on C-reactive protein, which is accepted as a marker of inflammation.

Moncada: Whether you are affecting the inflammatory process independently or you are affecting something which follows platelet aggregation is impossible to tell from that type of experiment, isn't it?

Oliver: To complete the story about Macmillan. It is true, as Gus Born and Duncan Thomas have pointed out, that his *Nature* paper was the first one to show the second phase. All I did was to get hold of a Born aggregometer and give him a minute amount of lab space. We then published another paper, which was not about the second phase. Poor Macmillan, a tense man, committed suicide and so the theme did not continue.[118]

Prentice: I think there is uncertainty on the question of aspirin dose and inflammation. Charles Warlow looked at two different doses of aspirin in his stroke study – 300mg and 1200mg. We found that there was no difference in the effect on bleeding time, which is quite clear.[119]

One point to add to Duncan Thomas's excellent account of the aspirin story. I think Harvey Weiss and Lou Aledort published in 1967 in the *Lancet* and, correct me if I am wrong, I think they were probably the first persons to show that ingestion of aspirin in humans prolonged the bleeding time by inhibiting platelet aggregation by collagen, and that correlated with the lack of platelet secondary response *in vitro* and a physiological effect in humans.[120] I think they were the first to show prolonged bleeding time with the aspirin patients and correlate it with collagen inhibition.

---

[117] Ridker *et al.* (1997).

[118] Professor Michael Oliver wrote: 'The noncontinuation of the research was my fault. I was a research fellow, working on my own on lipoproteins, and was wholly occupied with initiating what later became known as the WHO clofibrate trial. [Principal Investigators (1978)]'. Note on draft transcript, 5 May 2004.

[119] UK-TIA Study Group (1988); Hampton *et al.* (1990).

[120] Weiss and Aledort (1967).

Thomas: The effect of aspirin on the bleeding time had been known for some time. You are quite right, they did measure it, and showed it was prolonged by three minutes on average in their ten subjects. Even dear old Armand Quick of the Quick test did some studies with aspirin and showed that it prolonged the bleeding time.[121] Perhaps Weiss and Aledort were the first to look at it systematically.

Born: I think Clive Page's story is fascinating, because it's really an unexpected new function of platelets and opens up a whole new area to work on, which is what he does. I asked the question 'what happens in thrombocytopaenia?' and we now have to ask whether people who are thrombocytopaenic, for whatever reason, are more liable to infections. There are such people, of course. Have you any answer to that yet?

Page: I haven't, Gustav, but I think there are some interesting observations in the literature that people with asthma, when studied at post mortem, very rarely have, in my understanding from my reading, any evidence of calcification of major arteries compared with age- and sex-match controls. It's almost as though having atopy may be protective against having cardiovascular problems. Now I don't know how much of that has been looked into, but there are now several studies that people with an atopic phenotype have a prolonged bleeding time using the template bleeding time in the skin.[122] You can show that they also have a mild haemostatic defect, so it may be that in the case of atopy, this defect protects against cardiovascular diseases.

Harrison: I wanted to go back to the history of aspirin. Did you tell them about Dr Craven from Glendale, California? He was writing in the *Mississippi Valley Medical Journal*, which I don't peruse every week, and so many of us I think missed his claim, which was an interesting one.[123] He simply said that people who had their teeth out on aspirin bled a bit, it might stop you clotting a little. So he gave it to a lot of veterans he was responsible for and wrote a paper saying that nobody, and it's an interesting comment, nobody who religiously stuck to the dosage schedule had a coronary or cerebral thrombosis. This was an efficacy, not an intention-to-treat approach. We didn't know about that report when in 1971 we gave (I kind of invented the $n = 2$ trial) aspirin to a couple of patients with recurrent retinal platelet emboli and showed that

---

[121] Quick (1966). See biographical note on pages 153–4.

[122] Szczeklik *et al.* (1986).

[123] Craven (1953). See Appendix 2, page 85, for a facsimile copy of the paper.

you could switch them off. When you stopped the aspirin, after the appropriate number of days, the attacks returned. The interesting thing in the context of this meeting, is that we published the result even though it was only two observations, to advertise for cases for a trial.[124] Of course everyone said, 'Oh, I can give my patients aspirin' and referred no more patients to us.

Meade: I am glad you mentioned the paper in the *Mississippi Valley Medical Journal*,[125] because I was thinking about it and, as reported, the results seem quite striking. It's obviously not a controlled comparison, but nevertheless an early attempt to look at the aspirin story. What year did you say that was published?

Harrison: 1953.

Thomas: And it was 1500 patients, which is impressive – a prophet crying in the wilderness.

Meade: I think we should try to get the reference to that paper into the proceedings.

Moncada: I was going to say that the 1953 paper certainly is an important one. I have a copy of it and use it in my talks.[126]

Elwood: Craven wrote three papers, and two of them have already been mentioned, but I have copies of all three.[127]

Dr Y S Bakhle [Mick]: I just wondered, on a slightly philosophical note, as Duncan has just pointed out how several of these papers came together almost spontaneously, in a very short time. Is there a reality to the idea of 'due time', a time at which an idea suddenly becomes common and functional and accepted, or is that just romance?

Thomas: I agree with you, Mick, it is often people knowing each other. Don Chambers has referred to a group earlier, people like Marjorie Zucker and Harvey Weiss, who were in New York together.[128] The UK is small and everybody pretty well knows what's going on. I think you are right, but it's well to remember that people speak to each other, quite apart from the journals.

---

[124] Harrison *et al.* (1971).

[125] See note 123.

[126] See Appendix 2, pages 85–91.

[127] Craven (1950, 1953, 1956).

[128] Weiss (2003).

Meade: I think this phenomenon is sometimes referred to as synchronicity, and doesn't always involve people who know each other. Other scientific advances have been made, haven't they, in the same sort of way or have been developed quite independently by different people who happen to have arrived at the conclusion that that was the right thing to be doing.

Chambers: On the other hand, there is a whole literature developing, actually started by a molecular biologist by the name of Gunther Stent, on 'prematurity in scientific discovery'.[129] I have characterized this actually as the ligand–receptor argument for scientific acceptance, which postulates that the audience you are addressing has to be prepared to accept the new discovery, and thus your comment about Watson and Crick. The initial discovery by Avery, McCloud and McCarty of DNA being the 'transforming principle' was not accepted by the scientific community. To illustrate this, that discovery was made in 1943;[130] in 1950 DNA was not mentioned at all at a major international congress on genetics held in Berkeley, California.[131] The beauty of the Watson–Crick discovery utilizing model-building by Watson and the data of Franklin, Gosling and Wilkins, was that the structure of DNA looked right for its proposed function as the genetic material. Had the DNA that was studied by X-ray diffraction been derived from the bacteriophage phiX-174, which contains single-stranded DNA, the structure would not have been double-helical and there would be no base complementarity, and thus the characteristics presumed necessary for the double helix and the association with the DNA story might have been delayed. Chance, luck and acceptance are almost intangible qualities for good science.

Moncada: It is well known in science that when you look at a discovery with hindsight you can trace the background work that led to it. Usually there is an acceleration of the generation of information leading to the breakthrough. For

---

[129] Stent (1972). See a later evaluation based on papers from a symposium held at the University of California at Berkeley in December 1997 in Hook (ed.) (2002). See Reply to Gunther Stent, on the alleged 'prematurity' of the work of Avery, MacLeod and McCarty in Stent (1972) (submitted to *Scientific American*, but not published), No. 238 in the Oswald T Avery collection at http://profiles.nlm.nih.gov/CC/A/A/H/L/ (visited 21 February 2005).

[130] Avery *et al.* (1944). Oswald Avery's papers are held by the National Library of Medicine, Washington DC, as part of the Joshua Lederberg Papers, and available at http://profiles.nlm.nih.gov/CC/Views/AlphaChron/date/10002/ along with the freely available reprint at www.jem.org/cgi/reprint/149/2/297 (both sites visited 2 November 2004).

[131] Chambers (1995).

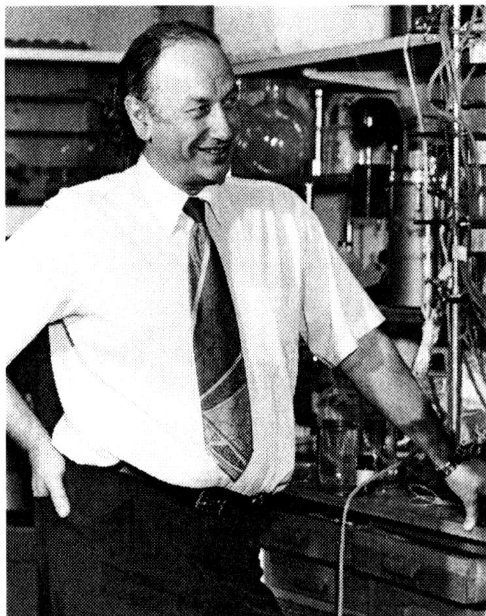

Figure 11: Professor Sir John Vane, c. 1986.

example, Watson and Crick did not arrive at their conclusions in a total vacuum – other people, including Linus Pauling,[132] were also close to it. Some, like Rosalind Franklin,[133] were there already.

Hunter: I would like to comment on what was said about synchronicity, when several people pay attention to the same fact in a short period of time. There is a completely opposite phenomenon for which there is no term in pharmacology, a drug which has a highly important therapeutic effect in fatal illness but is simply ignored. There are two examples of this: one is streptokinase, isolated in 1946, purified in 1953 and then ignored for two decades.[134] The other is metformin, an effective agent in the treatment of polycystic ovary syndrome (PCOS). I suggest that there should be a new technical term for this, using the analogy with obsolescence, which would be somnolescence.

---

[132] See the electronic resource, 'Linus Pauling and the race for DNA: A documentary history' [Corvallis, Oregon: Special Collections, Valley Library, Oregon State University, 2003] at http://osulibrary.orst.edu/specialcollections/coll/pauling/dna/index.html (visited 2 November 2004).

[133] Maddox (2002).

[134] See Glossary, page 166.

Born: Quite a number of years ago, John Vane, when he was Research Director of the Wellcome Foundation or even before, pointed out that when a pharmaceutical company was synthesizing analogues, the first was often the best and remained the best. I can't think of an example just now, I am sure other people can. The first analogue is often closest to the natural, endogenous substance, so that is another way of looking at this.

Meade: We won't go down that path just now. Are there any other comments on the topic we have just been discussing? I hope, Tilli, you won't mind that the last part of the discussion has been of a rather general nature about how some of these discoveries come about, but I think that's very interesting and very important.

Tansey: This is precisely the kind of interaction that we want to record.

Meade: Everybody has been very good about sticking to time, and actually there are one or two additional topics that people have suggested they want to bring up. We are very fortunate to have two of the key players in the prostaglandin story here today, Rod Flower and Salvador Moncada. Rod Flower, would you please start off the prostaglandin story?

Flower: I suppose it is difficult to know where to start, but since this is a historical occasion perhaps we could go back very briefly to the 1930s. Two very important discoveries were made at that time. George and Mildred Burr in the US were working on fatty acid deficiency in rats, and established that there were some fatty acids that were essential to life.[135] The other important discovery came from the early work of Ulf von Euler, who was probably the key player in the early development of prostaglandins.[136] He spent some time with Henry Dale and then with J H Gaddum, and during their time together, he discovered Substance P, and when he went back to the Karolinska Institute he took with him the knowledge of bioassay and he began to look at different tissues to see whether they contained Substance P.[137] I have got a nice quote from him here: he said:

> After my return to Sweden it seemed natural to continue my studies on tissue extracts in order to get some idea of the distribution and possibly the physiological role of the active

---

[135] Burr and Burr (1930).

[136] von Euler (1935, 1936). For more recent details on the effects of prostaglandins, see Morrow and Roberts (2001a): 669–80.

[137] See Harrison and Geppetti (2001). See also http://nobelprize.org/medicine/laureates/1970/euler-bio.html (visited 13 January 2005).

> factors occurring in the different organs....In due time and after several excursions, using a large variety of organ extracts including some from accessory genital organs from various animals, I decided to test human seminal plasma on the blood pressure of a rabbit. The effect of even a small amount was dramatic. The blood pressure of the rabbit dropped to very low levels, whilst my own probably went up some.[138]

Ulf von Euler was convinced at the time that he was dealing with Substance P again, but over the next couple of years he effectively ruled that out by showing that the substance he had was actually an acid and that it could be extracted into organic solvents. He then went on, just before the outbreak of the Second World War, to begin some analytical work, but unfortunately the war supervened. However, he had reached the point where he had discovered that seminal vesicles contained a very large amount of this bioactive material, and he had acquired a huge stock of sheep and bovine organs for his work. After the war when work resumed he opened the freezer, took them out, found they were still active, and this, I guess, was the foundation of the Karolinska Institute's work on the subject.

One interesting piece of trivia is that he initially thought he had identified this new hypotensive agent in the prostate gland and so called it 'prostaglandin'. It turns out that he was mistaken because the anatomical book he was using was incorrect, and it was actually the vesicular gland he was using. He later wrote:

> In retrospect it would have been better to name them vesiglandin A and B, since both were prepared from the vesicular gland, or its homologue, the seminal vesicle.[139]

After the war, work resumed. By the early 1960s, he was using a brand new technique – mass spectrometry[140] – which was, I think, probably only available at the time in two labs in the world, one of which was the Karolinska Institute. They were able to identify the structure of two prostaglandins, which they called E and F, because of their relative solubility in ether and phosphate buffer (phosphate begins with F in Swedish). At that time no one really understood

---

[138] von Euler (1982): xxxi.

[139] Ibid.

[140] For another application of the then emerging technique of mass spectrometry, see Tansey and Christie (1997): 78–9.

how these compounds were synthesized, although by the early 1960s they had already been infused into man, and the infusion of prostaglandin E caused a very sharp fall in arterial blood pressure, headache, and, rather ominously I thought, an oppressive feeling in the chest. I am not quite sure what that was due to. By the mid-1960s, the Karolinska group as well as a group at Unilever in The Netherlands, who were also very active in the field, had elucidated the way in which prostaglandins were synthesized and had identified the nature of the reaction. Today the enzyme that converts some essential fatty acids to prostglandins is called cyclo-oxygenase, but in those days it had other names.[141]

The whole area of prostaglandin research owes a lot to bioassay, and platelet aggregation, also occupies a very unique position in the whole prostaglandin story. I will just mention a couple of important findings. One is the description in 1969 by John Vane and Priscilla Piper of something called rabbit aorta-contracting substance (RCS).[142] This was a very labile substance which was released from perfused organs, particularly the lung, in response to various stimuli, and which contracted the rabbit aortic strip very sharply. This was to prove to be a very important observation in the whole field. As they began to explore the RCS phenomenon, John Vane's group noticed that you needn't have the perfused organ, but you could generate RCS if you infused crude microsomal extracts of cells which were known to contain the cyclo-oxygenase enzyme. Later Richard Gryglewski, working with John Vane, reported in a paper:

> This result was interpreted to mean that the process of prostaglandin biosynthesis includes RCS as an intermediate and that, once formed, RCS can spontaneously give rise to a prostaglandin.[143]

What they had noticed was that in fresh preparations the RCS disappeared very quickly, but as it did so the prostaglandin content went up and they concluded that one thing was disappearing and giving rise to another. The discovery of RCS in 1969 provided the immediate backdrop to the whole aspirin story.

If I can just digress again for a second or two. There were lots of explanations for aspirin's action around at the time. Most of them were really wide of the

---

[141] See Morrow and Roberts (2001b).

[142] Piper and Vane (1969). See also Hamberg *et al.* (1975).

[143] Gryglewski and Vane (1972): 456.

mark, but since this is a historical occasion, we should mention Harry Collier's contribution, because he had already described aspirin as an 'antidefensive drug', because it could counteract pain, fever and inflammation. He made the observation that aspirin could block broncho-constriction caused by bradykinin, and he thought that perhaps there were receptors for aspirin, and he actually called them 'A receptors', the A standing for aspirin. Later on, he abandoned this idea, and he wrote instead in one of his reviews that aspirin acted:

> rather by inhibiting some underlying cellular mechanism that takes part to different extents in the different responses mediated by different endogenous substances.[144]

One of those phrases that rings down the years.

So to 1971. Of course everyone knows the story of aspirin. The starting point was that John Vane's group were looking in the arterial circulation of anaesthetized dogs for RCS, and they found that it was released into the arterial circulation when the lungs were mildly hyperventilated. They also noticed that if they gave the dogs aspirin first, then the RCS disappeared. John wrote:

> While I was writing a review paper, including the results of these experiments, a thought occurred to me that perhaps should have been obvious earlier on: in all these experiments (and those of many other workers) the 'release' of prostaglandins must in fact amount to a fresh synthesis....That is, prostaglandin output in these experiments, although very low...was still far higher than the tissues' initial content of these hormones. Evidently, then, the various stimuli...which released prostaglandins were in fact 'turning on' the synthesis....A logical corollary was that aspirin might well be blocking the synthesis of prostaglandins.[145]

As we all know, he tested this in 1971, using cell-free extracts of guinea-pig lung,[146] and at the same time Sergio Ferreira and Salvador Moncada published a paper in the same issue of *Nature*, showing that the action of aspirin and indomethacin blocked prostaglandin generation by perfused organs.[147] Joe

---

[144] Collier (1969): 372.

[145] Vane (1972): 64.

[146] Vane (1971).

[147] Ferreira *et al.* (1971).

Collier and I also demonstrated at the same time that oral aspirin reduced prostaglandins in human seminal plasma.[148]

I want to mention again one of those odd episodes of synchronicity: also working in John and Gus's department, although apparently unaware of these developments, were Bryan Smith and Jim Willis. They were interested in the effects of aspirin on platelets and their hypothesis was that aspirin inhibited platelet aggregation by inhibiting the secretion of phospholipase A1 from platelets when they aggregated. They did a very simple but elegant experiment where they gave human volunteers 600mg of aspirin, took the platelets after an hour, added thrombin, and found that phospholipase levels were not changed, but prostaglandin levels were dramatically reduced. Their paper on the action of aspirin on platelets and prostaglandins went into the same edition of *Nature* at the same time as John's paper.[149] So the aspirin story began.

A couple of other things about the role of platelets in the prostaglandin story: one is that platelets played a key role in establishing the fact that prostaglandins are important in human physiology. This came about because the Karolinska scientists discovered a family that had a bleeding tendency, and this was discovered to be caused by platelet cyclo-oxygenase defect and they found that these platelets could not be found to aggregate with arachidonic acid, but they could be made to aggregate by adding back the endoperoxide intermediates that Samuelsson and his colleagues had discovered.

The next part of the story was trying to identify what Vane's RCS actually was and, as I have said, Samuelsson's group came up with the idea that there was a labile intermediate in the synthesis of prostaglandins.[150] The half-life of this intermediate, which was prostaglandin G_2, was actually much longer than that of RCS. They employed a very clever technique using platelets, whereby they added prostaglandin G_2 to platelets and they noticed that there was a time delay in the kinetics of aggregation, and that during this time another intermediate accumulated. This intermediate was subsequently identified as thromboxane A_2, and turned out to have exactly the same half-life as RCS, and so the identity of Vane's RCS was finally established. Again, I will just mention Jim Willis, because his work is not widely known, I think partly because he did all his research at night when everybody else was away, and during the day he

---

[148] Collier and Flower (1971).

[149] Smith and Willis (1971).

[150] Hamberg and Samuelsson (1974).

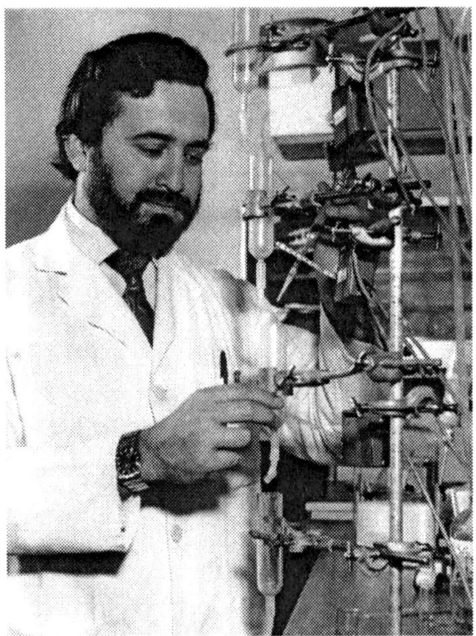

Figure 12: Dr Salvador Moncada performing a cascade bioassay, 1986.

spent most of the time servicing his Allard, of which he was very fond. But he did do some seminal work and he was one of the first to describe the generation by seminal vesicle enzyme of a substance that aggregated platelets very rapidly. He called this factor 'labile aggregation stimulation substance' (LASS). And he had also done, interestingly enough, an experiment where he injected this into mice and found that it killed the mice, because it caused intravascular platelet aggregation. He pursued this idea, but eventually it got lost in the torrent of other papers that subsequently appeared, which is a shame, because I think it was an important observation.

I don't really want to say any more, because I know Salvador will have a lot to say on this subject as well, particularly about the discovery of prostacyclin. I would stress that platelets have been integral to the whole prostaglandin story, and to the discovery of these labile intermediates thromboxane A_2, the endoperoxides. The discovery of the family with the missing cyclo-oxygenase was crucial in determining a role for prostaglandins in physiology and I would be happy to answer questions afterwards.

Meade: Thank you very much, Rod. That's exactly the sort of thing we wanted to hear. I will now ask Salvador Moncada to give us his recollections and interpretations of the other aspects of the story.

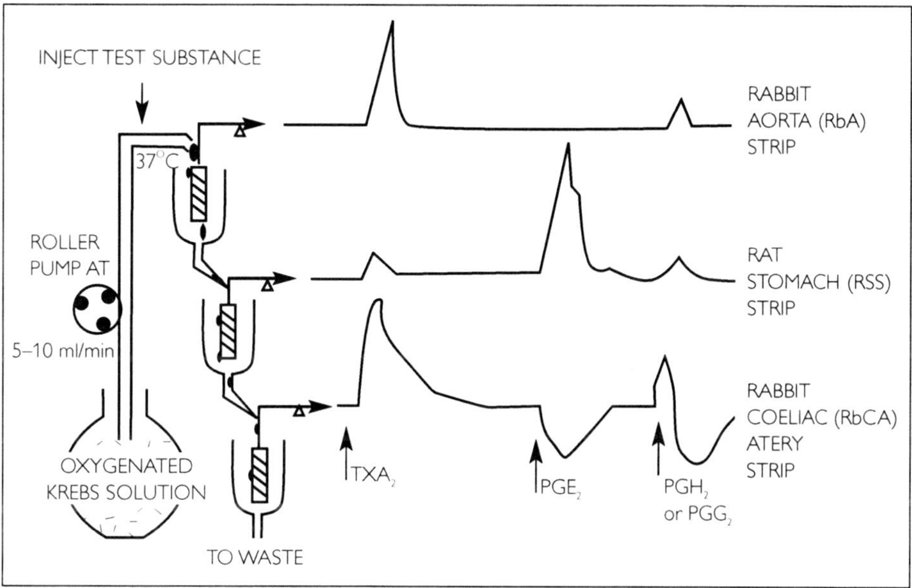

Figure 13: The technique of cascade superfusion. Warmed, oxygenated, physiological saline trickles sequentially over a bank of tissues. This experiment demonstrates the formation of a novel prostaglandin that relaxes rabbit coeliac artery, from the endoperoxide precursors PGG_2 and PGH_2.

Key: PG (prostaglandin); TXA_2 (thromboxane A_2).

Reproduced with permission, from Vane (1992), *Animal Experimentation and the Future of Medical Research*, 46. © Portland Press Ltd.

Moncada: The story as far as it concerned me started in early 1971 when I joined John Vane's group at the Royal College of Surgeons. At that time, coming from a medical background, I didn't have any experience in research, and I was starting from the very beginning. But in the very first few weeks, I learned to do the cascade bioassay, in John Vane's style, and one of the first projects he asked me to do was to hang several tissues on the cascade [see Figures 12 and 13], put arachidonic acid onto them to see whatever response they produced and then look at the effect of aspirin. Almost immediately it was clear that arachidonic acid was producing responses in tissues which could be blocked by aspirin-like drugs. That was already confirming some results that John had obtained using lung homogenates and doing biochemical measurements of prostaglandin synthesis. Because of those results, John invited me to join him and Sergio Ferreira in doing experiments in the dog spleen *in vivo*. We showed that catecholamines release prostaglandins from the spleen and that aspirin-like drugs inhibited that release. That work ended up as one of three papers that we published in 1971.[151]

For the next three years Sergio Ferreira and I spent most of our time trying to elucidate the meaning of these observations in relation to pain and inflammation. This led us to the conclusion that the prostaglandins were not really acting as mediators of inflammation and pain, but they were modulating the response of mediators such as bradykinin. So aspirin-like drugs were not blocking the process of inflammation, but were taking away this prostaglandin-based amplification process. I left the Royal College of Surgeons after finishing my PhD and went back to Honduras for a year. In 1975 I came back, this time to the Wellcome Foundation. John Vane had moved from the Royal College of Surgeons to be Director of Research at Wellcome and he had invited a small group of people to join him. We went with Rod Flower, Gerry Higgs, Geoff Blackwell and Sergio Ferreira to start setting up the laboratory at Beckenham, Kent.

On my way back from Honduras I stopped at the Florence meeting on prostaglandins where Bengt Samuelsson presented the results on thromboxane A_2. It was a fascinating story, as you heard from Rod Flower, and was closely connected to the work of Piper and Vane on rabbit aorta-contracting substance (RCS). For this reason, when I arrived at Wellcome we started a project trying to identify whether there was a separate enzyme that was responsible for the generation of thromboxane A_2. We started to do experiments in which we used the prostaglandin endoperoxides as possible substrates for a second enzyme in the platelets. We did this work with Phil Needleman and Stuart Bunting, and found such an enzyme, which we called thromboxane synthase, that was responsible for the conversion of prostaglandin endoperoxide to thromboxane A_2. We also identified the first inhibitors of this enzyme, namely imidazole and some of its analogues. The imidazoles had been described to have different actions, including effects on bleeding time. Because of that, among the many other compounds that we tested, we tried the imidazoles, which turned out to be very good selective inhibitors of thromboxane synthase and were the starting point for the pharmaceutical industry later on to develop inhibitors of these enzymes. The results were published in *Nature* and this time we published in collaboration with Bengt Samuelsson and Mats Hamberg from the Karolinska Institute, who had supplied the prostaglandin endoperoxides.[152]

---

[151] Vane (1971); Ferreira *et al.* (1971); Ferreira and Moncada (1971). See also Vane (1992).

[152] Bunting *et al.* (1976); Needleman *et al.* (1976); Moncada *et al.* (1977).

Towards the end of this project we thought that it would be worthwhile mapping the distribution of the thromboxane synthase in the body. We started to do a systematic study; however I was specifically interested in the vessel wall for several reasons. The first was that I was always thinking about platelet–vessel wall interaction and not just platelet aggregation *per se*. The second reason is that Sergio Ferreira and Fernando Ubatuba in our laboratory were trying to develop a measurement of bleeding time in the rat by superfusing the tail and measuring the amount of haemoglobin in the fluid with a photocell. Surprisingly, in some of these experiments the bleeding time was arrested very rapidly, suggesting vasoconstriction, rather than formation of a haemostatic plug. This made me think that the vessel wall might also be making thromboxane A_2. So, when Richard Gryglewski joined us for a sabbatical, I suggested to him a project looking for the formation of thromboxane A_2 in the vessel wall. We looked for thromboxane A_2 and for the classical prostaglandins using an enzyme preparation from pig aorta together with the bioassay cascade. We found that there was indeed an enzyme in the vessel wall that was metabolizing the endoperoxides, but the product, whatever it was, was not thromboxane A_2 or any of the known prostaglandins that we could detect by bioassay. And that was the beginning of the discovery of prostacyclin, which we started to call PGX [prostaglandin X or PGI_2].[153] We knew we were generating a substance that relaxed the vasculature, but so did prostaglandin E_2(PGE_2). We managed to distinguish between PGX and PGE_2 using a strip of bovine coronary artery, which fortuitously contracts to PGE_2 but relaxes to PGX. At some point we thought that PGX might be HHT [12(S)-hydroxy-5Z,8E,10E-heptadecatrienoic acid], a known metabolite of prostaglandin endoperoxides, but this turned out not to be the case. The breakthrough came by chance in a discussion with Stuart Bunting and Richard Gryglewski over a cup of tea. I said that we had been looking for thromboxane A_2, which is a vasoconstrictor and a proaggregating substance, and we might have found exactly the biological opposite in the vessel wall. Stuart Bunting and I tested the idea that same afternoon and we found that, indeed, whatever we were making from the vessel wall was probably the most potent inhibitor of platelet aggregation that had been described – about 50 times more potent that PGE, as we calculated it. That is the story of how we discovered prostacyclin.[154]

Meade: Which is what this is about, so thank you, Salvador.

---

[153] Originally described as an unstable substance (PGX) in Moncada *et al.* (1976).

[154] Vane (1983).

Born: I don't know if I am allowed to make this remark, but considering the number of people who are here who were in my department at the College of Surgeons at that time, I would just like to say that it was an amazing heyday, with both the platelets and the prostaglandins, and Bryan Smith and Salvador and Rod, Lawrence Youlten and Nicky Begent, and many others. So, it ought to be pointed out and kept on record that it was a remarkably good time. Yesterday, Bryan Smith sent me his historical sketch of the time which I can make available.[155]

Meade: Yes, I think that's a very important point.

Professor Sir Christopher Booth: The College of Surgeons was very active in researching in John Hunter's time. I don't know what their contributions have been in recent time, but what was it about the College of Surgeons that produced that remarkable laboratory at that moment?

Born: It's a good question. I hadn't thought about it quite like that. I got there in 1960 as Professor of Pharmacology in succession to Bill Paton. John Vane was already there as senior lecturer. We had been friends, John and I, for nearly ten years and our friendship continues to this day. There was an easy-goingness; we were very open and totally at ease with everybody, and if anybody was difficult, we soon cured them.

Meade: I think we should say that it's a pity that John Vane isn't here, and I am sure that we would all like to send him our very best wishes.[156]

Thomas: May I just add a comment to what Gustav said, as one who spent a year there? It was a remarkable department. I think the surgeons didn't really know what they had, but they appointed some outstanding people. That's what it boils down to, it is the people, not the College of Surgeons as such.

Meade: We will tell the College what you have said.

Hunter: This is a relatively small point, but the man who triggered off all this activity was Lord Webb-Johnson, and he insisted that there should be proper scientific training for people before they took the Fellowship of the Royal College of Surgeons (FRCS), and this led to their having research interests there. Lord Webb-Johnson approached the Royal College of Physicians, so

---

[155] Professor Bryan Smith died on 24 March 2005. For the historical sketch, see Smith (2004), and for an obituary, see Ashby *et al.* (2005).

[156] Professor Sir John Vane died on 19 November 2004. See Moncada (2005).

that the Royal College of Surgeons could be in the same place, could share laboratories, and the Physicians, I am ashamed to say, refused.

Bakhle: Might I make a comment about the bioassay system.[157] I think that what is very important is that both thromboxane A_2 and prostacyclin are short-lived, and what's even more important, they decay to biologically inactive products, so any bioassay process that requires extraction, an extract and then testing, would have given you a nil result. I think that was the power of what we, at the College, had. We had this semi-instantaneous assay system that would demonstrate, immediately as it was generated, some sort of biological activity. What Samuelsson[158] at the Karolinska Institute in Stockholm had was a fantastic analytical mass spectrometry system which could only work obviously on extracts, something which had decayed, and so *he* couldn't detect biological activity, and *we* couldn't detect structure. It was this curious thing, we, the department, had to demonstrate that there was an activity there to look for, and by the time that Samuelsson had got to it, of course, the activity had gone. You had to work backwards from the stable compound, from 6-oxo-$PGF_{1\alpha}$, or from thromboxane B_2, to what the activity might have been, which, of course, was done, but what was interesting was this dichotomy of abilities.

Moncada: Certainly that's one of the great things about the bioassay system, and I don't think that all these discoveries could have been made at the time they were made, if it hadn't been for the flexibility of the bioassay system. I remember the first experiments with trying to measure thromboxane A_2. It was so labile that, in order to detect any activity, we had to put the enzyme on ice to slow down the breakdown of the biological activity generated. With a half-life of 30 seconds or less, it was incredibly difficult to work with. However, I always think that the experience we gained working with thromboxane A_2 was extremely useful when we began to work on endothelium-derived relaxing factor (EDRF)/nitric oxide (NO), which, as you know, is even more unstable.[159]

Flower: Could I just add that the short-lived nature of these compounds, specifically prostacyclin, was one of the problems that led us to look for a way of measuring platelet aggregation in blood, which didn't necessitate us spinning

---

157 See Vane's Nobel lecture, Vane (1983).

158 Professor Samuelsson's Nobel lecture, 'From Studies of Biochemical Mechanisms to Novel Biological Mediators: Prostaglandin endoperoxides, thromboxanes and leukotrienes', is freely available at http://nobelprize.org/medicine/laureates/1982/samuelsson-lecture.html (visited 23 February 2005).

159 Palmer *et al.* (1987).

blood for 20 minutes to get the PRP. That's how we came initially to develop the whole-blood aggregometer. It was specifically designed so that we could infuse prostacyclin into animals or people, take blood samples and straight away measure the antiaggregatory response without having to go through a preparative phase where often the effect of short-lived intermediates was lost.

Professor John Dickinson: Can I ask how the funding of that famous laboratory came about? In other words, how many full-time people were paid by the College of Surgeons, not to do anything very specific, but to foster research, to teach young surgeons its own methods? One can see how once the great discoveries were made, people joined in, and all sorts of grants came in. But are we saying three, six, ten full-time staff, got the whole thing off the ground?

Meade: Gustav, what's the answer to that?

Born: I have to think rather hard. The College of Surgeons paid[160] for my chair from the Vandervell Endowment, and for John Vane as a senior lecturer; and we had two other lecturers, John Thompson and John Gardiner. So there were four academic staff by the College, plus technicians, who were permanent and our most delightful cleaner, Scotty Fenn, who became a close personal friend and godmother to one of our children. That describes the atmosphere I think. We attracted many grants. From the time I came to the College in 1960 I headed the Thrombosis Research Group of the MRC until John and I left in 1973. John attracted a lot of money, but I am not quite sure now – I don't want to be inaccurate – where that came from. We were pretty well funded for that period.

Meade: That's a very good answer to the principles at any rate, and we can perhaps fill some of those points later. John Hampton, while we are on the subject of funding, you were going to say something about that anyway.

Hampton: When I was listening to the other presentations, and thinking what happened when I was young and doing all this, the funding wasn't really an issue, because the universities were much wiser. They appointed the best guy they could get to head a department and they gave him a senior lecturer, a couple of lecturers, a technician, and a washer-upper, and told them to get on with it. Whereas now, if you are lucky, you get the chair and you are on your own.[161] And I think the result is obvious. I have children who are doing PhDs

---

[160] For the background of the Department of Pharmacology at the Royal College of Surgeons, see page 163.

[161] For a discussion of unsupported chairs, see Reynolds and Tansey (2000): 28, 59.

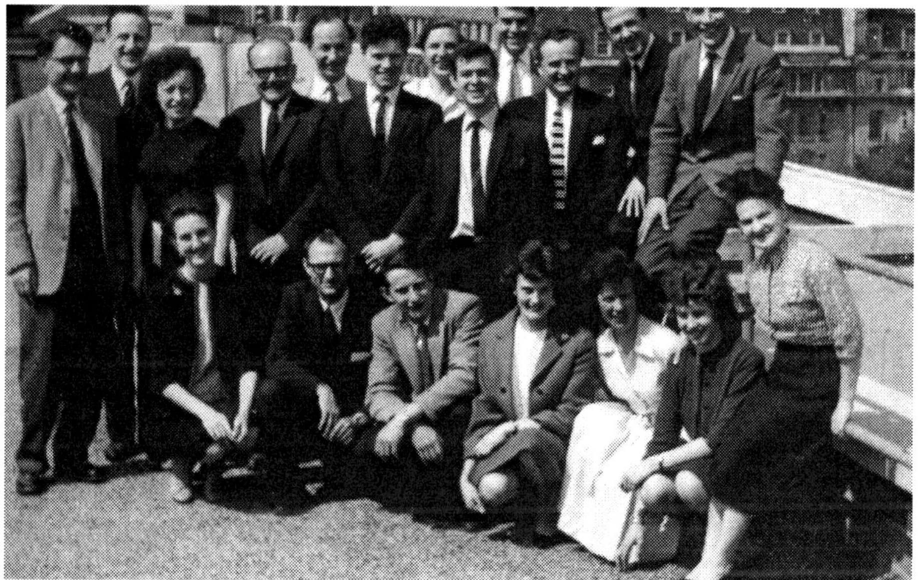

Figure 14: Royal College of Surgeons' Laboratory, *c.* 1963.
Standing, L to R: Gustav Born, John Thompson (lecturer, later Professor of Pharmacology at Newcastle), Olive Nialls (Professor Born's secretary), Durwood Smith (visiting Professor of Pharmacology from Vermont), John Vane (senior lecturer, later personal chair, Nobel Laureate, 1982), John Haynes (technician, who moved to Newcastle with John Thompson), Michael Cross (co-worker of Professor Born killed in 1964 aircrash),[162] Victor Clark (technician), Peter Gorinski (technician), Zigi Sabikowski (workshop mechanic who built aggregometers), Domenico Regoli (from Lausanne, Switzerland, co-worker of John Vane), Geoffrey Langston (chief technician), Scotty Fenn (Mrs Isobel Mills-Fenn, departmental cleaner). Sitting, L to R: Shirley Cross (wife of Michael Cross, later Mrs James Sherwood), Oleh Hornykiewicz (co-worker of Professor Born from Vienna, Austria, who later discovered the dopamine deficiency in the brain of Parksonian patients), Derek Nichol (technician), Margaret Day (research student), Anne Stockbridge (Margaret Day's technician), Sue Glover (Michael Cross's technician).

---

[162] On their way to the Second Conference on Blood Platelets at Oak Ridge National Laboratories, Oak Ridge, Tennessee, Michael J Cross, Philip A Geisler, Alfred Leitner and Robert H Levin, were among the 39 killed when their United Air Lines flight to Knoxville, TN, crashed in the Great Smoky Mountains on 9 July 1964. Professor Donald Chambers wrote: 'Ted Odell Jr and M Baldini organized this conference with the aim of bringing together platelet researchers from across the seas. Although the meeting did accomplish this purpose, its success was marred by the terrible plane crash in which four participants, including Mike Cross and Al Leitner, were killed. The organizers debated whether to call the meeting off but wisely concluded it was best to continue as a memorial to our deceased comrades.' E-mail to Mrs Lois Reynolds, 6 April 2005. For 'In Memorium' and abstracts of papers presented at that meeting, see Hollaender and Freireich (1965); and for two obituaries of Mike Cross, see Anonymous (1964); Born (1964b).

and they will not go into the academic world, because they see how you have to fight every inch of the way for funding, and they say that it's not worth it. I think everything we have been hearing today really depends on the time when wise men appointed other wise men and let them do their best. There was a phase of MRC funding: Tony Mitchell had a ten-year MRC grant for the set-up at Nottingham, but that all went, and the MRC lost interest in anything that didn't have a molecule attached to it. As for the role played by industry, it is interesting that for all the things we have heard about earlier, industry hardly came into it. We had a little bit of industrial money in Oxford and then Nottingham from Boehringer relating to *Persantin®* (dipyridamole) and its relations. To the best of my knowledge, aspirin didn't have any industry money. And the industry didn't get interested until we had clopidogrel and the CAPRIE study,[163] which I was involved in, which was US $250 million for one clinical trial. Then, of course, they got interested in the 2B3A antagonists, and goodness knows how many noughts are on the end of the grants for that. But I think it is interesting that everything we are talking about was done on an old-fashioned funding system.

Peart: I had the unfortunate task of spending four years of my life helping the College of Surgeons to run down the Institute in 1992.[164] It is a sad thing to say, but that's the truth of it. The College actually put a lot of money into the Institute, it changed it's name of course to the Hunterian Institute, but there were a lot of chairs, and there were many extremely good people in the Hunterian Institute. But there was always this imbalance between the surgeons and the research that was going on. The teaching was relatively easy, in the sense that anatomy, physiology and even ophthalmology had their chairs, and there were some eminent anatomists and physiologists who held those chairs. So there was a lot of tradition, and yet that tradition was not enough to help the Institute survive, because the amount of money required just could not be found from the College of Surgeons' finances. For example, you have got to remember that Down House, Charles Darwin's house in Kent, was actually rescued from dereliction by a surgeon, Sir Buckston Browne, and there was a very large animal facility there.[165] I should think there were not less than 500,

[163] CAPRIE Steering Committee (1996).

[164] Professor Peart was Master of the Hunterian Institute, Royal College of Surgeons of England from 1988 to 1992. For further details of the history of the Institute, its records, and the subsequent closure, see www.aim25.ac.uk/cgi-bin/search2?coll_id=263&inst_id=9 (visited 27 January 2005).

[165] For a description of the RCS's research institute from 1931 to 1989, known as the Buckston Browne Research Farm, named after the surgeon Sir Buckston Browne (1850–1945), see note 164.

which were being used to produce a dental vaccine. I was never too keen personally on the idea of a dental vaccine, but there it was and it had to be shut down because it was too expensive to run.

The tradition that I clung to in pharmacology and physiology was to keep something going that kept running. There was even a department of biophysics, an extremely good department, which I moved to the Institute of Child Health, because I felt it deserved to be perpetuated. Of course the staff fought very hard for their existence, and very successfully, because they continued to produce lots of extremely good work. Priscilla Piper has been mentioned already. But it's to the great credit of the College of Surgeons that the Institute survived as long as it did.

Meade: I think we will have one final comment from Gustav and then we must move on.

Born: I was going to suggest moving back to a platelet topic again. John Hampton mentioned dipyridamole as a drug, *Persantin*®. This is an interesting short story, from the time we were working on various inhibitors. One of them was dipyridamole as inhibitor of adenosine uptake by platelets and red cells in order to increase its potency as a platelet inhibitor. I had a lovely lady called Dinah James, an Englishwoman, working with me for a year. She was Professor of Pharmacology from Ibadan [Nigeria], an authority on African trypanosomiasis, and she told me that trypanosomes cannot make purines *de novo*. They have to take up purines from the tissues. So we thought, 'Let's try dipyridamole and see if we could stop the uptake of adenosine by trypanosomes.' We did that and published a paper on it in *Parasitology*,[166] showing an effect. I said in the 'Afterword' review that I didn't know whether anybody took this further, or I would have heard about it.[167] It turns out that Peter Richardson [present in the audience] went to the Internet (about two years ago) and found that there were 33 papers based on our finding. In other words, something that had happened with platelets has become a big story in African sleeping sickness, and which is still going on. At least two colleagues are working on this in Britain, Professor Keith Gull in Oxford and Professor Simon Jarvis in London.[168]

---

[166] James and Born (1980).

[167] See Born (2002a).

[168] See Born (2003a). Professor Peter Richardson provided a list of the citations to James and Born (1980), dated 8 May 2002, which will be deposited along with other documents and tapes from the meeting in Archives and Manuscripts, Wellcome Library, London.

Meade: We may have a chance for some sort of general discussion at the end and, Peter [Elwood], you might comment on that, but I think we must move on now to the whole question of aspirin and the prevention of thrombotic disorders. Peter Elwood is going to introduce the topic on the arterial side. Then Colin Prentice is going to discuss the venous side and then we will have further discussion.

Elwood: May I say first of all that in her invitation to this meeting Tilli Tansey said that among the questions she asks are: 'How is research funded and why?' 'Who are the influential individuals and groups involved, for example, a lab technician?' I would like to state that if I say 'I' or 'me', do record it as 'we', because there is a whole team behind everything that I say.

May I mention Lawrence Craven again, because in his first paper (which was not published in the *Mississippi Valley Medical Journal)*, he makes a lovely point that women take aspirin rather often for their pains and aches, while men tend to scorn such an 'effeminate' remedy.[169] Craven went on to wonder if this difference might explain the sex difference in the incidence of heart attacks.[170] The bottom line of course is that despite the fact that he advised 8000 friends and patients to take an aspirin a day, Lawrence Craven himself died of MI.

There are obviously several strands in any trial, and that's certainly true of our first trial of aspirin and MI. But from our general reading of the literature, our interest in aspirin goes back I think at least to the mid-1960s, and at that time I suggested to Archie Cochrane, the Director of the MRC Epidemiological Research Unit (South Wales), that we set up a prospective study in which we would do tests of platelet function and test the prediction of subsequent vascular events. Then in the classical epidemiological fashion we would look for the dietary and lifestyle determinants of platelet function.[171] I went round the experts in this country and abroad, and there was no test of platelet aggregation which we judged at that time would be suitable for a large epidemiological study based on 2000 to 3000 men. Platelet aggregation in platelet-rich plasma (PRP) had been described by Gus Born and by John O'Brien, but we felt this test could not be done on sufficient numbers of men.

---

[169] Craven (1950) was published in the *Annals of Western Medicine and Surgery*. For an alternative interpretation of sex-specific use of analgesics, see Reynolds and Tansey (2004): 21–2.

[170] Craven (1950).

[171] See Ness *et al.* (2002): 53–7 and Appendix 1, page 81.

Later we did platelet aggregation in 2500 men in the Caerphilly study.[172] Professor Serge Renaud supplied his mobile laboratory, which was installed in the Caerphilly Miners' Hospital for five years. Andrew Beswick, who is with us today, did the aggregation tests, using PRP first of all, and later whole blood.[173]

But to go back to the aspirin story, we felt in the mid- to late 1960s that there was no test of platelet aggregation that we could do on a large enough cohort for an epidemiological study. So we suggested to Archie Cochrane that as a 'second best' we thought we would hit the platelets with aspirin. Aspirin was getting into the literature, and we were influenced among others by O'Brien's paper in 1968, in which he called for a trial of aspirin.[174] Harvey Weiss had called for a trial of aspirin.[175] So as 'second-best' to an epidemiological study, we suggested to Archie Cochrane that we set up an aspirin trial, and over the next few years we admitted 1400 post-MI patients and the results of that trial were published in 1974, the first randomized trial of aspirin.[176]

The results were in terms of total mortality. We were very exacting epidemiologists in those days and we felt that total mortality should be the index of success or otherwise, but although we didn't publish it, total incidence of MI did show a highly significant benefit of aspirin, but total mortality was not quite statistically significant. Nevertheless, the trial was published and it excited tremendous interest. By 1980 the results of six trials were published. We did an overview of those six trials on the back of an envelope and presented the results at meetings. Richard Peto picked this up and he presented a paper to the inaugural meeting of the Society for Clinical Trials, based on those six aspirin trials.[177] This gave momentum to the Society for Clinical Trials, and to the idea of doing overviews of all the relevant evidence. Now over 140 randomized control trials of aspirin and vascular disease have been reported, and a number of people have pointed out that aspirin is certainly the most well-established and the most cost-effective prophylactic available in clinical practice.[178]

---

[172] Caerphilly and Speedwell Collaborative Group (1984).

[173] Elwood *et al.* (2001).

[174] O'Brien (1968b).

[175] Weiss and Aldort (1967).

[176] Elwood *et al.* (1974).

[177] Anonymous (1980); Hennekens *et al.* (1988).

[178] Antiplatelet Trialists' Collaboration (1994).

As the Chairman mentioned at the beginning, aspirin is now of interest in cancer and other conditions, but that's not a topic of this meeting. Some of the things that I have learnt today from Clive Page and others would give a possible mechanism for that reduction of cancer risk by habitual aspirin-taking.

When we published our paper, we were aware of two other studies: one was by Breddin, who did studies of platelet aggregation, but using a different method. He had a rotating glass container, which he rotated and watched the platelets aggregate. We surmised that CO_2 was probably being driven off from the plasma and the platelets were aggregating because of the change in pH. Breddin set up a randomized trial of aspirin, but it was a very small and rather flawed, published very shortly after our trial.[179] The other study was by Hershel Jick,[180] who conducted a study of hospital patients, questioning them on what drugs they had taken before they came into hospital. He questioned them on about the third or fourth day after admission.[181] He got a whole series of diagnoses, and he looked at the matrix with many hundred cells, searching for unknown relationships between diseases and drugs taken before admission for various conditions. The one thing that stood out in his table like a sore thumb was a very marked negative association between taking aspirin before admission to hospital and a confirmed diagnosis of MI. He immediately realized that there were two explanations: one was that aspirin was protective and people who took aspirin were not coming into hospital with MI. But the other explanation was that aspirin taken in the prodromal period before an MI was killing patients, and people who had taken aspirin didn't survive to be questioned on the third

---

[179] Breddin *et al.* (1980).

[180] Dr Duncan Thomas wrote: 'May I just add a note about Hershel Jick's contribution to this story, because I think it exemplifies a theme we have mentioned already about personal interactions. Hershel and I worked in the same hospital in Boston, and one day in the late 1960s we were having lunch together. I had just returned from a sabbatical year in London, and had brought back the first Born aggregometer to Boston. I was enthusing to my companions about the remarkable effect of aspirin on platelet aggregation and a rheumatologist at our table remarked that it was a clinical observation among his colleagues that patients with rheumatoid arthritis on large doses of aspirin seemed to have a low incidence of coronary artery disease. At this point, Hershel Jick said he would go and look at his data from the Boston Collaborative Drug Survey to see how aspirin intake correlated with myocardial infarction, and of course he found a negative correlation. Subsequently, his group went on to report that regular aspirin use in 7496 controls was 5 per cent, but only 0.9 per cent in 658 patients with acute MI.' Letter to Mrs Lois Reynolds, 14 May 2004. See also note 181.

[181] Jick *et al.* (1970). The Boston Collaborative Drug Surveillance Programme started in 1966, co-directed by Hershel Jick and Dennis Slone.

or fourth day. That put him and us in an enormous dilemma. We were two-thirds of the way through our trial and we actually broke the randomization code. We felt that if aspirin was killing people, we wanted to know whether or not to continue our trial. We were much criticized later for breaking the code, particularly by Sir Richard Doll, but we felt that we just had to do it.

Meade: Thank you very much. That makes an excellent introduction and there will be lots to follow that later on. Colin, would you like to speak now for a few minutes about the effect of aspirin on the venous side.

Prentice: Thank you very much, Tom. I think for a time there was a thought that arterial thrombosis is platelet led and is reduced by antiplatelet agents and venous thrombosis is fibrin/red cell led, produced by thrombin. Therefore anticoagulants such as warfarin and heparin would be effective in venous thrombosis and the antiplatelet agents effective in arterial thrombosis. Well, the truth is more complex than this and as you have shown yourself, Tom, and as a number of Norwegian and Dutch studies have shown, carefully administered anticoagulant therapy after MI seems to be an effective treatment, and anticoagulants are in use in Holland and Norway, but not too much in the UK, because we use aspirin.[182] So there is a discrepancy there.

The venous thrombosis story really started when Rory Collins and his epidemiologists carried out the meta-analysis in 1988 in the *New England Journal of Medicine*, showing that if you took all the postoperative deep vein thrombosis prevention trials in which aspirin had been compared with placebo or heparin, there was at least a one-third reduction in deep vein thrombosis by aspirin and a 50 per cent reduction in pulmonary embolism.[183] We were discussing this, and Rory was lamenting the fact that most of the endpoints have been surrogate endpoints, that is radioactive-labelled fibrinogen-I^{125} or venography, rather than patients getting a swollen leg through deep vein thrombosis or falling dead with pulmonary embolism. I think the strength of the big studies using clinical endpoints was actually indicated by the streptokinase studies, and when two large studies were done showing that streptokinase reduced mortality after MI, it was used by virtually 100 per cent of doctors after that time.[184] The next stage of the story, I think, took place as

---

[182] Sixty Plus Reinfarction Study Research Group (1980); Smith *et al.* (1990); Meade and Brennan (2000); Meade (2001); Fasey *et al.* (2002).

[183] Collins *et al.* (1988).

[184] See Appendix 3, pages 93–112.

all the best things do, in the bar, and that was a tapas bar in Barcelona. It was during the XIVth Congress of the European Society of Cardiology [1992] and Mike McMahon from Australia was there. He had been in discussion with Rory Collins, an epidemiologist, and Anthony Rogers, also from Australia, and they said in view of Rory's and my interest in doing a clinical endpoint study, why didn't we get together and do a big prospective study, rather like Peter Elwood had done many years previously?[185] Which is essentially what we did, and in the year 2000 we published the Pulmonary Embolism Prevention (PEP) study.[186] We looked at 13 500 patients having surgery for fractured hip, divided randomly into placebo or 150mg aspirin a day, starting preoperatively, and continuing for 35 days. To cut a long story short, using clinical endpoints with an independent clinical judging committee, the incidence of clinical deep vein thrombosis (DVT) was reduced by over one-third, the incidence of pulmonary embolism by almost half, and the incidence of fatal pulmonary embolism, which is the thing that interests most patients postoperatively, was reduced by almost 60 per cent. So we had a very similar picture to the heparin story and I think this is where the situation rests. It looks as though aspirin is an effective agent clinically after surgery, to prevent pulmonary embolism and deep vein thrombosis. Heparin is also an effective agent in this situation, just as in MI, so that both aspirin and anticoagulants appear to be effective agents.

I think the only sad thing is that it's difficult to combine two effective agents, because then you run the risk of untoward haemorrhage, and it always brings us back to the point that we are looking at haemorrhagic risk versus thrombotic benefit.

Meade: Thank you very much. As you say, the idea that aspirin might affect venous thrombosis was really not accepted, certainly not in this country, for a long time, until the developments that you described came about. Of course, all the interest in aspirin has now led on to primary prevention trials, in other words trials in people who have not yet had an event, but who might later on. And by and large the results of those trials have been similar to the secondary prevention trials, but they are important, because secondary prevention trials can only be done on the people who survive. Since a very high proportion of people who have their first coronary event die in that event, it is obviously

---

[185] See Appendix 1, pages 81–4.

[186] Pulmonary Embolism Prevention (PEP) trial (2000).

important to see what happens in those who have so far remained free of clinical coronary disease. But of course these trials have their problems, because the incidence of the event is much lower. There's also the problem now, in both primary and secondary prevention, that aspirin can be purchased over the counter, and I suspect that there are a lot of people taking aspirin who don't realize that, particularly in primary prevention, the balance between the benefit and the risk is not as obvious as most people assume it is. In other words, there's a fairly low benefit to be set against a not insubstantial risk. There have now been five primary prevention trials, and they are being looked at in an overview by Colin Baigent in Oxford, and I think they will probably be published in an overview sometime in the next year or two. As far as coronary disease is concerned, I think the answer is very much the same as we have been hearing so far, but why is it that aspirin appears to reduce nonfatal events to a much greater extent than fatal events? That I think is a fairly consistent finding from both secondary prevention trials and particularly from the primary prevention trials. Salvador, you've got the answer.

Moncada: I think that it is because we may be looking at two different problems. The hypothesis that platelets might be playing a role in the developing atherosclerotic plaque, slowly aggregating on the vessel wall, is one thing. Aspirin might well have an effect on this process. However in the final event, when there is plaque rupture, many proaggregating substances are involved, including those that are not inhibited by aspirin. Then the possibility of affecting this with aspirin is less likely. That's what I would venture as a hypothesis. If you were to design an ideal antiplatelet agent for an *in vivo* effect it would be difficult to improve on aspirin. It acts at very small concentrations for as long as the platelets are in the circulation and it probably acts on platelets in the presystemic circulation, thus sparing the vessel wall. So, for prevention of the development of the plaque, if platelets are involved, aspirin might be the ideal drug.

Meade: Part of the story is the decline in what people regard as the required dose of aspirin. People were using gram amounts to begin with, as we have heard several times this afternoon already, and now I suppose 75mg or 100mg, not more than that, is probably what most people would consider effective and obviously safer than the larger dosage.

Moncada: The studies of Carlo Patrono are very clear.[187] If what we are intending is to inhibit thromboxane formation, then 75mg are good enough.

---

187 De Caterina *et al.* (1985); Patrono *et al.* (2001); Capone *et al.* (2004).

You don't need any more than that dose, since it will specifically and selectively block thromboxane A_2 formation and the second wave of platelet aggregation. The clinical trials seem to support the fact that a small dose of aspirin really works and that the pharmacological action can be linked to a therapeutic effect.

Thomas: May I just ask you a question, Tom? You rightly pointed out the pros and cons of taking aspirin, and that it is a fine balance, but I thought you had shown that it is in people who are hypertensive that the risks outweigh the potential benefits. Did I get that wrong?

Meade: We showed that people who are hypertensive didn't derive any benefit. They didn't actually experience any additional risks, but they didn't benefit. The people who derived the benefit seemed to be the people who are normotensive. A lot of these questions are going to be settled more firmly and more conclusively when Colin Baigent's overview comes out soon, which I think will be very important in terms of indicating who should or should not be taking aspirin.

Moncada: Do you know what doses of aspirin were used in those five trials?

Meade: There has been quite a wide range. We used 75mg in the Thrombosis Prevention Trial. The Physicians' Health study used 325mg on alternate days.[188] Richard Doll's trial in the doctors' study used 500mg a day.[189] So the answer is that there has been a wide range of doses.

Moncada: This is important to determine since as you increase the dose of aspirin the risk of side-effects increases. Let me remind you that at very high doses aspirin also has a certain fibrinolytic effect and this has not been discussed yet.

Meade: Over tea Alison Goodall mentioned to me the question of aspirin resistance, which is receiving a lot of attention at the moment. Is there such a thing as aspirin resistance that is actually any different from the fact that not everybody responds totally to almost any medicine, or is it something that is really a feature of aspirin?

Professor Alison Goodall: I was making the point from two perspectives. One is a reflection that, just at a time when data coming out from both primary and secondary prevention trials really do demonstrate that aspirin is effective, we

---

[188] Physicians' Health Study Research Group Steering Committee (1989); Hennekens and Eberlein (1985).

[189] Peto *et al.* (1988).

seem to be getting rather negative comments in the literature about the effects of aspirin, both in terms of the bleeding risk and aspirin resistance.[190] I think this reflects the haemostatic balance. If we go back to the points that were being discussed earlier about the platelet response in relation to disease progression and risk, there's clearly a wide range of platelet response in all populations. The data from populations that are post-MI, and from prospective studies all seem to be indicating that there is a very wide range of platelet response. This comes back to comments by Professor Born and Professor Moncada that the overriding event, which is plaque rupture, may subsume any antiplatelet effects of aspirin. This raises the issue of whether we should be perhaps now considering treating the individual rather than the population, because I think the approach until now has been to use one dose across the population. Maybe we are moving towards dosing that is related to the individual in relation to the level of their platelet response, which does appear to be consistent within individuals, and possibly also inherited.

The other point in terms in of aspirin resistance, is whether this phenomenon really does exist. I think the jury is definitely out as far as that is concerned [**Moncada**: Can you tell me what you mean by aspirin resistance?]. Aspirin resistance, as I understand it, has been defined in two ways. One is in epidemiological terms, looking at events in subjects who are on aspirin. There's conflicting data in the literature that suggests that in patients on long-term aspirin (this particularly seems to be associated with elderly patients with cerebral vascular disease) both the incidence of cerebral vascular events and the platelet response to agonist stimulation seem to decline over time. But there is an equal body of data suggesting that that doesn't happen. The other area that has become of immediate interest in the literature is a so-called aspirin resistance during or postsurgery. And there's a very open story there as to whether it's linked to some kind of expression of COX-2 in the platelets.[191]

Moncada: Quite. This brings us back to a previous point. Do we want to treat the platelets, in which case aspirin is ideal, or do we want to treat the vessel wall, in which case an anti-inflammatory action would be better? The complication of inhibitors of COX-2 is that the vessel wall makes prostacyclin using this enzyme and this might be the origin of the suggested 'vascular side-effects' related to the use of these drugs.

---

[190] Hankey and Eikelboom (2004).

[191] Zimmermann *et al.* (2001); Payne *et al.* (2004).

Peart: May I just say that surely the dose must be very important, and the variability of 75mg requires a bit of analysis. If you follow the reason for the introduction of 75mg by Garret FitzGerald, it was so that there was a small amount of aspirin which affected the platelets flowing through the gut, the vascular system.[192] And that the larger doses, as I am sure a lot of people here will say, affected the vessel wall. So you have got two pharmacological effects here. Do people still actually believe that what FitzGerald said was the case? It seems to have stood the test of time, and you must take account of that, surely, in so-called resistance, because the drug that has to go through the gut wall must be subject to all sorts of variables in that aspect.

Heptinstall: Very briefly, I believe that 'aspirin resistance' is difficult to define. For some it means that some people still get events while they are taking aspirin. On the other hand we have looked at hundreds of blood samples from people taking aspirin and I can categorically say that you get inhibition of thromboxane synthesis in everybody. Fullstop. I would make just one addition to that. I think Salvador said that he felt that 75mg produced good inhibition in everybody. I think on one occasion we looked at a blood sample from a lady with pregnancy-induced hypertension, and we did not see complete inhibition in that case. We had to increase the dose to get complete inhibition of thromboxane synthesis.

Meade: Just one more comment from Salvador. This discussion is getting too scientific and not historical enough.

Moncada: I was just going to repeat the comment that I made before. The evidence for platelet sensitivity versus vessel wall lack of sensitivity to aspirin is clear from many different experimental and clinical data. The evidence that all inhibition of platelets might actually occur in the presystemic circulation is also clear. And the inhibition of platelet aggregation by aspirin is permanent, while inhibition of the vessel wall, if it occurs, is short-lasting. That's why I was saying that if we ever thought about a drug to inhibit platelets, we couldn't have invented it better.

Meade: That's a reassuring note on which to move on to our last topic. This is, of course, to do with one of the other effects of platelets, and that is in the question of bleeding. That is obviously related partly to the aspirin story, which we have been hearing about, but there are other aspects of platelets that affect the bleeding profile of some patients and which have quite an interesting historical background. Peter MacCallum is going to tell us a bit about that.

---

[192] Charman *et al.* (1993).

Dr Peter MacCallum: Thank you, Tom, for asking me to say a few words about this. I hope others will pick up the baton when I finish. I think I am probably fairly unique in this symposium, being the only person who has made no contribution at all to the subject I am going to speak about. So, I can't give you any sort of inside information on historical advances, but others may well be able to contribute.

When we think about bleeding problems and platelets, we really divide them up into two broad categories: those that are caused by deficiencies in platelet numbers, thrombocytopaenias; and those that are caused by defects in platelet function. Compared with the other subjects that we have been hearing about this afternoon and the immense work that's been done in the UK over the last 40 or 50 years, and reading through the literature in preparation, when I was asked to talk about this topic, it appears that there has been a smaller contribution from British scientists to the hereditary aspects of platelets than there has been to prostaglandins, aspirin and other aspects of platelet biochemistry.

Sticking to the brief of British haematologists, as far as I could, talking first about thrombocytopaenia, of which the most common cause by some margin is immune thrombocytopaenic purpura (ITP). There's one cause of this condition where there has been a substantial UK input. Although the majority of the problems that we see with ITP are bleeding related, the condition I'm thinking of more commonly causes a thrombotic problem. This condition is called the antiphospholipid syndrome (APS), a name that has emerged over the last ten or 15 years to describe a problem that was first recognized back in the 1960s when Walter Bowie, a UK graduate who spent his career at the Mayo Clinic, Rochester, Minnesota, described the presence of a coagulation inhibitor in patients with systemic lupus erythematosus (SLE), which appeared to be associated with a thrombotic problem:[193] a paradox of abnormal coagulation in the test-tube with clotting in the patient and occasionally with thrombocytopaenia. And in the late 1970s and early 1980s, Graham Hughes at St Thomas' Hospital, London, was instrumental in introducing a test for this particular condition by identifying cardiolipin antibodies[194] [cardiolipin being derived from an alcohol extract of bovine heart mitochondria that was a component of the original Wassermann reaction (WR) reagent used in the syphilis test and was responsible for the false-positive tests for syphilis

---

[193] Bowie *et al.* (1963).

[194] Hughes (1993).

sometime found in these patients]. The St Thomas' unit, among others, has been important in furthering our understanding of a condition in which patients develop an antibody-mediated process that leads to a prothrombotic problem. That's one aspect of thrombocytopaenia which has a UK contribution. Another comes from the haematology department at the Royal Postgraduate Medical School, Hammersmith Hospital, London, where Sir John Dacie,[195] a very eminent haematologist from the 1940s through to his retirement in 1977, was very instrumental in setting up a group of haematologists who made an immense contribution to UK haematology.[196] In particular, he described and took forward our understanding of another condition that can give rise to thrombocytopaenia and also to thrombosis, called paroxysmal nocturnal haemoglobinuria (PNH), where again, as you sometimes see in the anti-phospholipid syndrome, both thrombocytopaenia and thrombotic problems occur. So thrombocytopaenia and thrombosis can clearly coexist. The group at the Hammersmith have been instrumental in identifying this and wrote a very significant paper, I think probably the world's largest collection of a very rare condition, in the *New England Journal of Medicine* in 1995.[197] Interestingly the causes of death in these patients was of interest – they had a series of 80 patients, 60 of whom had died, including about 15 deaths from thrombotic events, and ten from haemorrhagic events in relation to thrombocytopaenia – another significant UK contribution.

Moving on to disorders of platelet function I think there are one or two people in this audience who've described platelet abnormalities in the context of common medical conditions, in which platelet function is impaired and haemostasis is a problem. Duncan Thomas described problems of platelet function in patients with liver disease, if I remember rightly, and George McNicol and Stuart Douglas likewise for scurvy, back in the 1960s.[198] When one comes to discussing hereditary disorders of platelet function then a lot of the eponymous conditions come into textbooks and I don't think that the UK contribution has been so significant here. Glanzmann's thrombasthaenia was

---

[195] Professor Sir John Dacie died on 12 February 2005.

[196] Dacie (1979). This is an abridged version of paper read to the History of Medicine Section, 7 February 1979, including a brief outline of the contributions of Rickard Christophers, Peyton Rous, and Winifred Ashby.

[197] Hillmen *et al.* (1995). Platelet transfusions should be given when appropriate and long-term anticoagulation therapy should be considered for all patients.

[198] Thomas *et al.* (1967); McNicol and Douglas (1967); Thomas (1972).

described by a Swiss paediatrician, Bernard–Soulier syndrome by two French haematologists, Chediak–Higashi syndrome, a problem of dense granule secretion, by a Cuban and a Japanese, and Hermansky–Pudlak syndrome, by two Czechs, a range of very exotic names to a number of very rare conditions. In the coagulation field, as opposed to the platelet field, deficiencies of coagulation factors, haemophilia in particular, clearly aided the understanding of the coagulation cascade.[199] In contrast, and perhaps it is because these conditions are much rarer, it is not clear to me that the eponymous conditions of the hereditary platelet dysfunctions actually aided understanding of platelet biochemistry, and the recognition of the glycoprotein receptors and granules, but others may have different views.

Prentice: A question arising from the issue of haemorrhagic aspects and platelets. For many years the International Society of Thrombosis and Haemostasis (they might still be doing it) were looking at post mortem examinations of patients with von Willebrand's disease and haemophiliacs, because the positive side of having a platelet defect might be that you get less atherosclerosis and thrombosis. I am just enquiring from the audience whether any of those studies were completed or whether it was too difficult to find enough subjects for this study. Does anyone know the answer to that? [**Meade:** No, I think not]. I suppose now there's going to be so much treatment for these patients that the opportunity to study them in the sort of untreated state has been lost.

Goodall: One comment in relation to the contribution of the UK's haematologists to the study of rare inherited platelet disorders, and that is the name of Roger Hardisty.[200] Perhaps it is worth noting that I got into platelet research because Roger and I had a joint Wellcome Trust grant back in the 1980s to study the weak agonist response defect. Roger made a magnificent contribution to the understanding of all the rare platelet disorders.

Heptinstall: May I tell you just a very short story? Some years ago we wanted some platelets from a patient with Bernard–Soulier syndrome, because we had an antibody that we wanted to test to see if we could detect Soulier's syndrome by flow cytometry, and indeed we were able to do that.[201] The patient was a gentleman called Alfred and he was 80 years old. As we were taking blood and

---

[199] For disorders of platelet function, see, for example, Hardisty (1977). See also Tansey and Christie (1999): 45, 79.

[200] Hardisty (1983).

[201] Debre *et al.* (1952).

obviously we were chatting to him, it intrigued me that a man with a bleeding problem should live to the age of 80. In conversation he told us that he had a twin brother who died as a child from bleeding after a tooth extraction. That shows how a situation can manifest itself differently in different people, even in twin brothers. But the interesting story, coming back to aspirin, is that Alfred had a painful back. We talked about this, and I said, 'I don't suppose your doctor gives you any aspirin as an analgesic, given the fact that you have got Bernard–Soulier syndrome?' He said, 'Absolutely right, my doctor has always said I should avoid aspirin. I should never take any aspirin for pain.' So I said, 'Well, what do you take?' His answer was indomethacin.[202]

Meade: Peter, would you put disseminated intravascular coagulation (DIC) into this category of rather anomalous situations where a low platelet count could also be associated with a thrombotic element?

MacCallum: Yes, I would, and also thrombotic thrombocytopaenic purpura (TTP) and heparin-induced thrombocytopaenia (HIT). There's a whole host of conditions.

Meade: And who described those first of all?

MacCallum: Well, TTP was described by Moschcowitz in the 1920s.[203] DIC was described by a number of workers in the 1950s, while the term DIC was probably first coined by Hardaway and McKay. A number of clinicians were involved in defining HIT, but the original description was by two US surgeons, Weismann and Tobin, in 1957.[204]

Meade: It is interesting that this is a group of rather anomalous conditions where a low platelet count can also be associated with a thrombotic risk.

Oliver: Are we going to see more haemorrhagic events, with the increasing consumption of very long-chain fatty acids and fish oils? I would predict we are. The more consumption of dodocosahexanoate and pentanoate acids by those who are taking aspirin, it is likely that there will be more haemorrhagic events.

Meade: Ask the younger epidemiologists in ten years' time and they may be able to tell you. We have got one or two other topics that people have alluded

---

[202] For a discussion of the effects of indomethacin on platelet function, see Morrow and Roberts (2001b): 705–6. See also note 151.

[203] Moschcowitz (1925); McCarthy *et al.* (2004).

[204] Weismann and Tobin (1958); Hardaway and McKay (1959).

to or asked me about over tea which I think it may be nice to come back to. First of all, Peter Richardson, are there any further comments you want to make on the trypanosomiasis or dipyridamole stories?

Professor Peter Richardson: I think in the interests of time, it is better to defer the trypanosomiasis–dipyridamole story to another occasion, as it is a bit complicated.[205] I think it might be better to get to the other topic, artificial organs. The advent of blood-handling artificial organs presented a big clinical challenge, which only a few people get to see directly, but nevertheless it has been a considerable challenge. The pivotal timepoint, for example, for artificial kidney use for dialysis is 1961, with the invention of the percutaneous shunt by Belding Scribner in Seattle, which allowed for repeated connection of an artificial kidney to the circulation.

Cardiac surgery was being developed in the early 1950s, and increasingly it relied on evolving technology to provide manufactured components to be in contact with flowing blood. Denis Melrose in the UK was first to describe elective cardiac arrest to improve conditions in open-heart surgery.[206] The American Society for Artificial Internal Organs was initiated with a small meeting in 1954. Blood oxygenators for cardiac surgery were initially filtering devices, supporting blood in direct contact with oxygen, then disposable bubble oxygenators were made possible with the advent of defoaming chemicals. Dialysers intrinsically require membranes between blood and dialysate, and a California-resident Briton designed a highly successful membrane-based blood oxygenator, which was used by J Hill in San Francisco, not only in surgery but also in the first clinical attempt at multi-day support of a chest-trauma victim with acute loss of adequate respiratory function. The designer was M L Bramson, better known as the engineer who, in the 1930s, made a positive assessment of the prospects of Whittle's proposal for the jet engine.[207] His analysis of Whittle's project led to it being developed in the UK. His oxygenator design used 6m^2 of silicone-rubber membrane, and required fresh, sterile assembly on site prior to use, therefore lacking the convenience of disposable units. Other designs were developed, using typically less than half that area of

---

[205] Professor Peter Richardson has provided a list of the references mentioned by Professor Born (see note 168), which will be deposited along with the other records of this meeting, held in GC/253, Archives and Manuscripts, Wellcome Library, London.

[206] See Taylor (ed.) (1986). See also Dempster *et al.* (1968).

[207] Hill *et al.* (1972).

expensive membrane material in disposable units but having a higher bloodflow resistance and, in many cases, a higher tendency to problems with thrombosis although the blood was typically heparinized during use in bypass.

And so a big effort had to be made to study the materials, the junctions of materials, and various design and manufacturing processes that would diminish the extent of thrombosis.[208] And this took place largely within the aegis of the Artificial Heart Programme, part of the US National Institutes of Health, run at the time by Frank Hastings, who unfortunately died of a stroke at a rather critical time. Because the artificial heart itself was not showing much promise (there were big thrombotic problems, embolization problems, associated with it) there was a need to get some useful science into this. I think the critical piece in this was a paper, which was produced and published in *Nature* in 1970, by Nicky Begent and Gustav Born, who made studies of the effect of bloodflow rate on thrombo-stroke.[209] The experiments were intravascular, they were performed in venules, and they provided extensive quantitative information about thrombus growth, exponential in time as you increase the blood flow rate the exponential coefficient increased with blood flow rate up to a maximum, but then diminished as you went to higher blood flow rates. Understanding some of the consequences of that behaviour was very important in being able to design channels successfully in artificial organs that diminished the prospects of thrombosis being a clinical problem.[210]

It has got to the point where if you don't hear much about it, then it's not a major presence in the literature. There will be, I think, a reflection on this in the coming year, 2004, because it is the 50th anniversary meeting of the

---

[208] Professor Peter Richardson wrote: 'Leininger's group published on nonthrombogenic plastic surfaces in *Science* in 1966 [Leininger *et al.* (1966)], Kwan-Gett on thrombogenic areas in artificial hearts in 1967 [Nose *et al.* (1967)], and Dutton *et al.* [(1968)] made direct microscopic visualization of initial thrombus formation on foreign surfaces in 1968, which helped show the importance of platelet adhesion as a precursor to thrombus formation.' Letter to Mrs Lois Reynolds, 27 May 2004.

[209] Begent and Born (1970).

[210] Professor Peter Richardson wrote: 'Various international meetings brought British and other researchers together, such as the joint EEC–US meeting on blood oxygenators in Rungstedgaard, 1975 [Zapol and Qvist (eds) (1976)], the meeting on cellular adhesion applied to thrombosis and haemostasis, Saint Paul-de-Vence, 1980 [summary of presentations deposited with records of this meeting in the Wellcome Trust Library], and the New York Academy of Sciences' meeting on blood in contact with natural and artificial surfaces, 1986 [Leonard *et al.* (eds) (1987)], for example.' Letter to Mrs Lois Reynolds, 27 May 2004.

American Society of Artificial Organs, and they are calling for abstracts of papers which will include historical reviews.[211]

Moncada: Is the reason that you don't hear very much about it because the problem has been solved, or because people don't recognize the problem?

Richardson: The problem has largely been solved by a combination of procedures. The whole preparation of a circuit for use in bypass is itself a skilled process – shall we say, acquired through experiment. The materials and the manufacturing conditions have been refined to the point where most of these organs don't have thrombus problems in the time in which they are used, and some of them are used for days. With a pumpless procedure for chronic bypass with an artificial lung, for example, I have seen 50 days of continuous bypass.[212]

Moncada: We used to collaborate with a surgeon, Donald Longmore, who used to say that the problem existed and it was serious, but was largely ignored.[213]

Richardson: It was discussed back then, and it's being discussed again, curiously enough. There were researchers who were seeking information in the earlier trials, which were not planned out very well. They gave intelligence tests to the patients before and after surgery, and very often the patients appeared to be more intelligent after the surgery. The theory then was that we caught them in a nervous state in anticipation of the surgery and they did not perform very well, but having survived the operation, they were much more comfortable with the testing.[214]

---

[211] The programme for the meeting held in Washington, DC, 17–19 July 2004, is freely available at www.asaio.com/clientuploads/pdf/preprogram.pdf (visited 14 April 2005).

[212] Barthelemy *et al.* (1982); Liebold *et al.* (2000); Conrad *et al.* (2001).

[213] For details of early work on heart transplant surgery in the UK, see Tansey and Reynolds (1999), and for Professor Longmore's work in particular, see pages 3–11, 17, 21, 26–33, 52–4, 64.

[214] Professor Peter Richardson wrote: 'Hlatky *et al.* [(1997)] comments that coronary artery bypass often leads to short-term cognitive dysfunction, whereas coronary angioplasty does not. Perioperative cognitive dysfunction usually resolves, although a subgroup of surgical patients may continue to exhibit long-term cognitive dysfunction. This retrospective study indicated long-term function is similar in both groups. Another issue which has been examined involves the possible effect of the possible neuroprotective role of hypothermic cardiopulmonary bypass (CPB). In an associated study [McLean *et al.* (1994)], a randomized trial of normothermic vs hypothermic CPB, the authors found deterioration in scores of tests of psychomotor speed but not of memory in the early postoperative period, and did not consider any neuroprotective effect of moderate hypothermia was demonstrated. On the other hand, a more recent British study [Millar *et al.* (2001)] points to influence of pre-existing cognitive impairment.' Note on draft transcript, 8 March 2005.

We tried to see what might be sent into the patients from the extracorporeal circuits that might lead to neurological deficits, by building an ultrasound device to examine the bloodflow being returned to patients.[215] It could detect bubbles, emboli, even small loose pieces of plastic. A company was formed to commercialize the technology, but it found a profitable niche in quality control in photoresist electronics manufacture, and in secondary oil recovery, and built no more units for heart bypass circuits.

I'll take this opportunity to mention that Marjorie Zucker and other haematologists were much involved with groups examining blood-materials interactions.[216] I think her name was mentioned earlier, and I just thought I would make that link.

Harrison: For the last ten years we have been addressing this issue by neuropsychological testing patients before and after coronary artery bypass surgery. The change is not related to anxiety or depression levels. If you ask the patients, what they report is not accurate. You need to ask the spouse. There is real evidence of a decline in cognitive performance postcoronary artery bypass surgery, not in the majority, but in the minority of patients, and using that as an endpoint it has been possible to help the surgeons tighten up their technique, so that it is now getting increasingly rare. We hoped to use it as a model for neuroprotection, but as yet nothing has been found to act as a neuroprotective drug in this context. One of the problems now is that the incidence has fallen, and the studies are getting more and more difficult to do.

Meade: I think there's one more topic that I want to raise, and that's one that Stan Peart mentioned over tea, the question of retinal emboli.

Peart: Sorry to be talking so much. The thing that has always intrigued me about thrombosis is the way in which it disappears, and I noticed that there's not been much discussion about those sequences that follow thrombosis. You can't help but be impressed when you look at the retina – and I used to look

---

[215] Abts *et al.* (1978).

[216] Professor Peter Richardson wrote: 'She was a regular participant in the Columbia University Seminar on Biomaterials, and in connection with this an interesting paper is in a volume devoted to blood in contact with natural and artificial surfaces [Zucker *et al.* (1987)]. In this she and her colleagues seek to explain better the importance of the conformation of the von Willebrand Factor (vWF) molecule to the specificity of the glass-bead column platelet retention test being the only simple *in vitro* test that picked up vWF deficiency.' Note on draft transcript, 8 March 2005. See also notes 79, 107 and 128.

at them very frequently – and observe those little white emboli in the retinal arterioles and they would disappear in days or weeks. And, of course, we probably now believe that most of them come off the atheromatous plaques in carotid or other arteries. But this process also applies to much larger blood vessels. I mean in the early days of arteriography it was pointed out that quite extensive thromboses in the middle cerebral artery could actually dissolve and disappear. Therefore I don't think any discussion about what actually happens with platelets and the interaction with the vessel wall is complete without being able to try to explain that, because that's one of the other big variables, surely, in the subject we are talking about.

Meade: Has anybody got the answer?

Born: Of course, I haven't got the answer, but the process probably turns largely on things like nitric oxide. If the vessel wall hasn't been visibly damaged and you still have intact endothelial cells, then I don't know how it is in the retinal vessels, but the emboli come from down in the carotids, don't they? You are saying that they disappear and that there might be something different in the retinal vessels; or could it be some change in the origin of the emboli?

Moncada: I think what Gus Born is saying is probably right. We carried out many studies that remain largely unpublished, investigating the reversibility of platelet aggregation. The evidence suggested that *in vitro,* in the platelet aggregometer, the platelet aggregate can initially be dissociated by increasing cyclic AMP (cAMP) or cyclic GMP (cGMP); however, later on the aggregate becomes irreversible. Therefore, *in vivo* the clumps seem to be 'organized' very rapidly. I presume that the vessel wall is different since there the platelets are subjected to the actions of prostacyclin and NO throughout the process. I agree that this whole process is not understood very clearly.

Meade: To the extent that the platelet aggregate may also be bound up with fibrin, we shouldn't overlook fibrin deposition and fibrolytic activity as well.

Bakhle: Might I make a historical and a general point. At the same time as all the work on platelets was going on in the department, we had also stumbled on the idea that the endothelium was, biochemically, a very active cell. For instance, it clears 5-HT (5-hydroxytryptamine). Val Alabaster's PhD was on the clearance of 5-HT in the pulmonary circulation,[217] which was why Starling

[217] Alabaster (1971).

and Verney needed to keep the lungs in their perfused kidney circuits.[218] We also looked at the mechanisms of that clearance.[219] The other very important clearance function of the endothelial cells,[220] as Jeremy Pearson and I know, is that there are ecto-ATPases, -ADPases, and -AMPases, on the outside of the endothelial cells. So all those phosphates go down very rapidly to adenosine which actually can also be cleared by the endothelial cells. So I think what happens to the platelet is not just what the platelet is doing, but crucially how it interacts with the endothelium. And I think perhaps some of the divergencies that we have heard about between assays of platelet aggregation *in vitro* or *ex vivo* and what happens *in vivo* may be because at certain times what the endothelium is doing is crucial and may, if you like, overcome what the platelet is doing. So that now we hear about endothelial dysfunction as being a disease and perhaps being responsible for some of the cardiovascular effects of diabetes. And it's certainly true that in diabetics the output, I think, of NO, certainly of prostacyclin, from the endothelium is decreased. I think that the platelets story grew up in this atmosphere where we knew that platelet function could be affected by endothelial function. Now that, I think, was perhaps what Gustav meant when he said he didn't think that the aggregometer could necessarily predict clinical behaviour. That interaction between platelets and the endothelium was a background part of the department and is not obvious unless you were there at the time.

Meade: You have ended on a historical note, and I think that's where we should finish. We were beginning to make a very good case for a scientific meeting on the endothelium and all sorts of other things, which I hope the Wellcome Trust will take due note of. But we have come to the end of our

---

[218] Starling and Verney (1925). Dr Mick Bakhle wrote: 'This paper was written well before the identification of 5-HT in 1948 (Rapport *et al.* (1948)), but Starling and Verney discuss, at some length, various methods of maintaining a viable isolated kidney, incorporating a heart–lung preparation in the circuit. On page 325, they summarize their experience: "As soon as this [freshly defibrinated blood] reaches the kidney the vessels constrict firmly, so that it may be impossible to force a drop of blood through them. It seems that the defibrinated blood becomes 'detoxicated' in the heart-lung preparation, presumably in the lungs." (The inverted commas around detoxicated are S&V's own, not mine!) Although the serotonin (5-HT) used by Rapport *et al.* was derived from serum, a similar vasoconstrictor was also known to be present in defibrinated blood, from aggregated platelets in both conditions.' E-mail to Mrs Lois Reynolds, 20 April 2005.

[219] Alabaster and Bakhle (1970).

[220] Chelliah and Bakhle (1983); Gordon *et al.* (1986).

programme. I personally have enjoyed it immensely, I think it's been a very interesting one. Thank you all for coming, and to everybody for their contributions, particularly to the lead discussants. I would like to thank Gustav, who really was the organizer of this meeting, and the key person who thought that it would be a nice one to have, and also of course the Wellcome Trust Centre people who have given us an excellent afternoon in terms of the arrangements that they have made: Tilli Tansey, Wendy Kutner, Daphne Christie and Lois Reynolds. Thank you one and all, and drinks are now served.

Tansey: On behalf of the History of Twentieth Century Medicine Group, may I thank you all for coming and talking. It has been a great privilege to listen to you all. The work is not over, because we will be sending you the transcripts and we will be asking you to add, if you have anything else to add, to the transcripts; these can go as footnotes. Please also think about depositing your archives in the library here. This is not a ridiculous idea, we do want contemporary records in the library. And I would like to add the gratitude of this meeting to our Chairman. I think he has done an admirable job, so thank you very much.

Appendix 1

An edited and annotated extract from an interview with Professor Peter Elwood by Dr Andy Ness, 28 February 2001[221]

Caerphilly cohort study, 1979–ongoing

We had a post for a junior epidemiologist and it was largely looked on as a training post by the MRC, which had been awarded to a series of people, David Bainton and Ian Baker, for example. I advertised and we appointed John Yarnell,[222] a very bright person, who wanted to work on his own and he set up several studies. He did a bit of work on urinary incontinence, and then he put forward a proposal to look at high-density lipoproteins (HDL) in women. HDL cholesterol was a big item in the literature at that time, but almost entirely in men, and I thought, 'Yes, this is worth doing'. So he got a bit of money to employ four women and he set up a study in 800 women in Caerphilly.

I saw the potential in that study, and I urged John to set up a major heart disease study in men, testing a range of hypotheses and taking additional samples of blood, and asking additional questions to give a basis for testing new hypotheses which would come up in the future. It was always in my mind that any major study like that should always have the potential for testing new hypotheses.

If I can extrapolate just a little, it always seemed to me that epidemiology studies are so large and so unwieldy that they pick up a question like the relevance of HDL and it can be 10 or 15 years before any answers emerge. The answers are incredibly valuable, but by then the medical thinking has moved on and other questions have arisen, so any big epidemiological study has to be hung on one or two hypotheses in order to get funding. Those questions that the original study included are of very little value in the end, because the results take so long to emerge. If extra blood samples are taken, so that, retrospectively, new hypotheses which arise in the future can be tested, is a very necessary aspect of epidemiological studies.

---

[221] The full texts of the 15 interviews conducted by Dr Ness have been deposited along with papers and documents for the Witness Seminar, 'The MRC (South Wales) Epidemiology Unit', held on 23 March 1999, in Archives and Manuscripts, GC/253, Wellcome Library, London. Selections from some of these interviews have been published in Ness *et al.* (2002). See also www.epi.bris.ac.uk/mrc-caerphilly/ (visited 11 October 2004).

[222] See biographical note, page 156.

John put forward a [second] proposal to look at about 2500 men in Caerphilly. John Yarnell has always been given credit for setting it up and for doing a lot of the basic thinking and organization, and drawing up the sample, but I always insisted that it was a unit project, that we all had a part to play in it. And that's certainly how it turned out.

We all saw tremendous value in collaboration and so we drew in a number of people on lipids, on haemostasis. John O'Brien was one of the people, whom I collaborated with on aspirin and cardiovascular disease and he's very much a lateral thinker and so he was involved from the very beginning. He suggested a small package of haematological tests. Others, like Gordon Lowe in Glasgow, and then Rod Flower in Bath were drawn in later.[223] It was called the Caerphilly Collaborative Study, because I felt the real value would come from collaboration with men like Serge Renaud on platelets, John O'Brien on haemostasis, and Barry Lewis on lipids.

The involvement of other people in the unit was, of course, absolutely essential. Janie Hughes and Marion Jones looked after the records and the response rate. Marion followed up men who refused to come to the clinic, and offered to do the investigations in their home. I would take their blood, so we got the whole range of data from them. Without Marion and Janie, the study would have been an average, or below-average study, but they put in such a consistent effort without being asked, a product of their training over the years, in working with Archie [Cochrane] and others. It turned it into a very fine study, with a very high response rate, and a very careful documentation.

The study was launched in 1979, and it took four years to see the men, until 1983. John Yarnell chose the sample using the electoral register, and some of the doctors' lists. We wanted a complete sample of men within the age range 45 to 59 years of age. A questionnaire asked a few general questions, such as the age of the respondent, which was a key factor in identifying this particular age group within the community. Letters were sent to virtually every male on the electoral roll, in order to pick the sample, and get a complete sample between those age groups. We set up the study in church halls, the YMCA, and in doctors' surgeries, moving around the town, seeing people in the different areas. We had one dedicated person who visited the men to persuade them to come to the clinic, and there were six stations in the clinic where different tests

---

[223] Elwood *et al.* (2001).

were done. We piloted all this with my friends and contacts. Later, friends from church and the neighbourhood would ask me at intervals, 'Well, what's happening up in Caerphilly? You haven't had us up for a long time.' We timed everything and tried to envisage delays in the procedure so that men went through as smoothly as possible.

The record-keeping and other details were developed *ad hoc* as we went along, and one of the very, very big mistakes we made, which we bitterly regretted, was the use of numbers from 1001 upwards. It was discovered later that in the Speedwell study in Bristol, the same numbering had been used with an overlap in the numbers. I had always suggested within the unit that each research topic have a unique number – for instance our study on school children was 32s, 33s, and 34s followed by 01, 02, 03, for the different subjects. Janie and I developed this system to enable us to immediately identify the study from the number on the questionnaire. When Caerphilly was being set up, we just used straight numbers and got into a terrible situation later when the samples from Caerphilly and Speedwell were stored together, which has been very difficult to unscramble.

In those days a sample of 2500 wasn't particularly small. We would have liked it to be bigger, but I insisted that it should be intensive and that we should collaborate with as large a number as possible and add in as many tests as possible. For instance, at a later stage, we added in lead, arthritis with Silman,[224] and other things. It was a very intensive study and we were prepared to go on for a long time, rather than have large numbers.

South Wales was a very stable area. Some of the cohort studies in London and places like that [other large conurbations] got into trouble trying to follow up their sample. We knew that Caerphilly was a very stable area and we expected it to be a very long-term study. Initially we had thought of ten years, but I don't think we had thought of that as an absolute end to the study.

With regard to women, we were aware of the opportunity that we were missing in not looking at [both] men and women, and so towards the end of the study we added a sample of 250 women, but to my knowledge sadly nothing has ever been published about those women. When we started to analyse them – I took a personal interest in those 250 women – I looked at a number of things, but Peter Sweetnam pointed out the drift by the laboratory estimations. There was

[224] Silman (1986).

always a drift over time and the women came in at the end of the study, so we would either have to compare the women with the last 250 men in the Caerphilly sample, or we would have to indulge in some rather dubious standardization process to take account of the drift and the changes in the laboratories. It was so difficult. So, yes it is a small study, but I think we have gained in other ways in that we have contributed to a very large number of hypotheses and to discussions about a large number of topics. Because John Yarnell's main interest was in HDL cholesterol and he teamed up with Barry Lewis in London and with Colin Bolton in Bristol, we had very detailed measurements. We also put in the upper lipid proteins, which were very new in those days, and we could have made it a lipid study. Ten years later we had difficulty in publishing the results of this wretched HDL fractions 2 and 3, which had been done for us. They were 'old hat' people said; 'Those methods are not appropriate now', [especially as] the protein's not in HDL-2 and HDL-3. I think the haemostatic and thrombosis evidence, [along with] platelets [are] the most valuable areas within the whole of the Caerphilly studies.[225]

[225] Other findings include: men who drank more than a pint of milk each day reduced their risk of heart disease and stroke by 30 per cent, compared with those who drank no milk; middle-aged men with depression are over three times more likely to suffer a fatal stroke. See Ness *et al.* (2002), 127–9. See also, for example, Renaud *et al.* (1979); Elwood *et al.* (1991, 1998, 2003).

Appendix 2

Facsimile copy of Dr Lawrence Craven's 1953 article[226]

38 MISSISSIPPI VALLEY MEDICAL JOURNAL

EXPERIENCES WITH ASPIRIN (ACETYLSALICYLIC ACID) IN THE NONSPECIFIC PROPHYLAXIS OF CORONARY THROMBOSIS*

Lawrence L. Craven, M.D.
Glendale, California

CORONARY thrombosis is one of the principal causes of sudden death, prolonged morbidity, or permanent disability, and strikes especially often males in their late middle age, who to all appearances enjoyed the best of health. Ordinarily premonitory signs are absent, and it is therefore impossible to institute some form of specific preventive therapy. The possibility of general, nonspecific prophylaxis is hardly taken into consideration, and the medical profession tends to maintain a similarly fatalistic attitude toward episodes of coronary thrombosis as does the laity.

There can be no argument that any definitive plan of prophylaxis—specific or nonspecific—depends on continued research and a more complete understanding of the etiologic and pathologic aspects of coronary thrombosis. But in the meantime experiences which might have a bearing on the general prophylaxis of the disease may not be entirely without practical interest.

It should be pointed out that only ten years ago the prophylactic use of anticoagulants in the presence of impending venous thrombosis or following coronary occlusion was still considered to be hypothetic or controversial.[35] Nowadays sufficient experience has been accumulated to establish precise indications and dosages for this type of medication, which is well on its way to becoming a standardized procedure.

The value of anticoagulant therapy using heparin and dicumarol in the prevention of embolism and repeated coronary occlusion has been demonstrated beyond any reasonable doubt. Thus the question arises whether the salicylates, which have essentially the same effect as dicumarol, but are less powerful,[36] do not deserve a place in the general nonspecific prophylaxis of coronary occlusion. Because of their lesser potency these drugs can be more freely prescribed, and may prove useful if administered to subjects most likely to experience coronary thrombosis, before the first episode has taken place.

More particularly, the value of aspirin (acetylsalicylic acid) in the general prophylaxis of coronary occlusion is suggested by observations accumulated during the past seven years. Concededly, the effectiveness of any type of prophylactic treatment is difficult to prove, and this applies especially to a procedure aiming merely at nonspecific prevention. Observations on healthy subjects can never be made under strictly scientific conditions, and resulting figures are only within limits suitable for statistical evaluation. Such findings may therefore merely have the value of preliminary impressions, and will be substantiated or refuted by subsequent clinical research. But as long as the field of general prophylaxis of coronary thrombosis is still outside the limits of present-day research procedures, preliminary observations may still be of practical importance provided:

1. the measure is safe in all subjects and throughout the entire extended period of medication;
2. the observations are not in opposition to trend and results of clinical and experimental research; and
3. it is well understood that the findings were not arrived at under strictly scientific conditions.

Aspirin (acetylsalicylic acid) was suggested as a general prophylactic of coronary thrombosis to 1465 healthy male subjects, mainly between the ages of 45 and 65 years, who were overweight and known to lead a sedentary life. It is common knowledge that individuals of this type are more frequently and earlier in their lives exposed to the dangers of sudden episodes of coronary thrombosis. But the precise cause of such attacks cannot be ascertained with any degree of certainty, and it must be assumed that a multitude of factors contribute to the development of coronary thrombosis. Undeniably, atherosclerosis plays a considerable part, but even most recent authors on the subject[28] are unable to account for the occurrence of specific episodes which are described as spontaneous events. Despite all electrocardiographic observations, and findings at autopsy, the matter is far from being resolved. How could it otherwise be explained that many persons with advanced atherosclerosis of the entire arterial tree live to a ripe old age, and then die of something else than 'heart disease'. There must be other factors which enter into the picture and are responsible for 'heart attacks'.

It is in this respect of interest to note that the incidence of postoperative

* Third Prize, 1952 Mississippi Valley Medical Society Essay Contest

[226] Craven L L. (1953) Experiences with aspirin (acetylsalicylic acid) in the nonspecific prophylaxis of coronary thrombosis. *Mississippi Valley Medical Journal* 75: 38–44.

thrombosis in the presence of atheromatous lesions is very low. "Autopsies have shown coronary vessels narrowed to an almost pin-point lumen at the site of atheromatous plaques, without the occurrence of thrombosis."[20] The finding is tentatively explained through elaboration of antagonistic substances in areas of atheromatous fatty degeneration, and it is concluded that the composition of the blood occupies a place in the causation of thrombosis. With all due regard for the differences between postoperative thrombosis and coronary occlusion, such findings should caution against overemphasis of the rôle of atheromas in the causation of coronary episodes.

In the composition of the blood, hypercoagulability and a resultant tendency toward thrombus formation may well be of crucial importance. It has been experimentally demonstrated that a primary relationship exists between thrombus formation and the clotting mechanism of the blood.[9] However, observations as to blood changes accompanying coronary thrombosis are contradictory. Ogura and his co-workers[33] found no increased coagulability of the blood immediately after coronary occlusion, and concluded that accelerated coagulation does not seem to play any role in the causation of thrombosis, but is rather the result of thrombosis and subsequent tissue damage; yet, once acceleration of coagulation is present, it may lead to further coronary episodes. Similar results were reported independently by two other groups.[18, 28] Entirely different findings were obtained when prothrombin determinations were made in a group of patients as a routine laboratory procedure, and readings before and after acute coronary occlusion could be compared.[10] It was established that coronary occlusion did not occur before prothrombin time fell well below 70 per cent of normal. The series is too small to permit any far-reaching conclusions. But it is interesting that observations started before onset of coronary occlusion differ from those made immediately following the first episode. In any case clotting is essentially a physico-chemical process which is theoretically reversible, especially as long as the clot has not yet become organized.[23]

Anticoagulant Therapy

From the foregoing observations and considerations it might be assumed that development of coronary occlusion can be prevented through anticoagulant therapy. Indeed, long-term anticoagulant therapy is applied for an indefinite period in various types of cariovascular disease as a prophylactic step against future recurrences.[15] These conditions include phlebitis migrans, recurrent thrombophlebitis, and recurrent coronary thrombosis with myocardial infarction. Experience with long-term dicumarol therapy is at present still limited,[32] but it is felt that the regimen is feasible. It is not claimed that attacks of coronary thrombosis can be entirely prevented by that therapy, but patients who formerly experienced repeated episodes could be kept free of recurrences under constant dicumarol medication.[25]

The same line of reasoning as that underlying anticoagulant therapy for the prevention of recurrences of coronary occlusion can be applied to the general prophylaxis of first episodes of coronary thrombosis. It is, however, evident that medication with dicumarol is not feasible in healthy subjects who are only suspected on the basis of general observations of being prone to coronary occlusion. The problem would be entirely different if reliance could be placed on premonitory signs, warranting institution of a more specific therapy.

Dicumarol, while not being an expensive drug, is potentially dangerous. Its effect must be checked by frequent prothrombin time determinations, and not every laboratory is well versed in the pitfalls of these tests.[31] Heparin is not only expensive and at times unavailable, but also for other reasons not suited for long-term prophylactic medication. It is therefore fortunate that in the salicylates, and especially in aspirin (acetylsalicylic acid) we possess anticoagulant drugs of lesser potency, but inexpensive, easily administerd, and entirely safe if taken in small doses.

In fact, it was practical experience with the anticoagulant properties of aspirin which led to experimentation with this drug in the general prophylaxis of coronary thrombosis. Some seven years ago it was noted that in an ever increasing number of cases, and for no apparent reasons, tonsillectomy was followed by secondary hemorrhage. This was all the more surprising as during the previous 25 years delayed hemorrhages had been observed only in exceptional instances. Obviously a change in procedure was responsible for these late complications. About that time we had begun to recommend Aspergum, one stick half an hour before meals and one at bedtime, for its mildly analgesic effect. It was discovered that the patients who subsequently developed serious hemorrhages had in each and every instance not limited themselves to four sticks of Aspergum as directed, but had chewed about twenty sticks a day, in order to obtain continuous comfort. Since there are 3½ grains of aspirin in each stick of Aspergum, the daily intake amounted to 70 grains (4.5 grams) of acetylsalicylic acid. Although this dose is not excessive when compared with those prescribed in rheumatic fever and similar diseases, the effect is apparently increased in the presence of an open wound. Hemorrhages appeared between the 5th and 7th postoperative day, and were occasionally serious enough to require hospitalization. Laboratory reports showed a reduced prothrombin level, and in two instances the readings were so low that the technician suggested that the operation had perhaps been performed by mistake in hemophiliacs! Hemorrhages were easily controlled through administration of adequate doses of vitamin K, and no such incidents have been noted since Menadione (2-methyl-1, 4-naphthoquinone), 2 mg. daily, was prescribed simultaneously with aspirin.

These experiences with secondary hemorrhages following tonsillectomy were confirmed by findings in nine patients with troublesome epistaxis. In each instance the patient had taken large doses of aspirin over extended periods of time, and recurrence of nosebleed was prevented by merely stopping the use of salicylates.

Similar observations concerning acetylsalicylic acid as the probable cause of secondary hemorrhage were made by Singer.[43] He noted hemorrhagic inflammation of the soft palate in about thirty per cent of patients who had undergone tonsillectomy, with secondary bleeding in five to ten per cent of the total number of patients. Routinely 10 grains (0.65 grams) of acetylsalicylic acid were given three to four times daily for alleviation to postoperative discomfort. When this medication was discontinued no secondary hemorrhage or hemorrhagic inflammation of the soft palate occurred following tonsillectomy in a series of 75 patients. In Central Europe, aminopyrine (Pyramidon), a derivative of antipyrine, is used in preference to the salicylates, and hemorrhagic complications are very rare indeed. It should be added, however, that aminopyrine may produce other undesirable side-effects.[46]

Singer's observations were confirmed by Neivert,[30] who found that some subjects will react after 24 hours to a total daily dose of 2.4 grams of acetylsalicylic acid with elevation in prothrombin time, while in others it takes much longer until a significant response can be detected. Before going any further in the investigation of the hemorrhagic — or more correctly the prothrombinopenic — action of the salicylates it should be mentioned that Ersner and his co-workers[12] ascribed secondary hemorrhage five to seven days after tonsillectomy to complete cessation of salivary secretions; saliva has a definite effect on wound healing, and considerably decreases the blood coagulation time.

Secondary bleeding following tonsillectomy, and epistaxis are due to the fact that with sufficient lowering of the prothrombin content of the blood hemorrhages occur in areas which are exposed to trauma and stress.[9] According to one report[34] five instances of epistaxis, one of which severe, were observed in the course of massive salicylate therapy; bleeding occurred at time of most pronounced hypoprothrombinemia and stopped of its own accord when the prothrombin levels returned to normal, in spite of continued administration of salicylates.

As early as 1891[3] it was recognized that salicylic acid produces hemorrhage in the mucous membranes of some subjects, and results in frequent and excessive menstruation in certain females. But only much later was it shown that salicylic acid can affect the blood coagulation mechanism *per se*.[22] This effect, first demonstrated in rats, was then also established in man,[38] and it was found that among the salicylates aspirin has the highest potency as prothrombinopenia-inducing agent.[42]

Occasionally hemorrhages can be traced to aspirin with a high degree of probability. For instance, in a rather recent report[29] it was established that prolonged intestinal bleeding was due to acetylsalicylic acid taken at the rate of 3 grams daily. In this case all other causes of intestinal bleeding could be eliminated; homorrhages disappeared when the patient was hospitalized and taken off aspirin, but the various symptoms recurred as soon as he returned home and again started self-medication with aspirin, in order to control rheumatic complaints. Such severe toxic reactions, however, are rare. Nevertheless, cases are on record in which death has been ascribed to medication with acetylsalicylic acid.[11] In two cases of this type widespread hemorrhagic changes were demonstrated at autopsy all over the body, and particularly involving the brain.[1] Generally speaking, fatal salicylate intoxication seems to occur more frequently in children than in adults.[45] Sometimes it must remain doubtful whether abnormal response to a compound containing aspirin should be traced to idiopathic hypoprothrombinemia, or whether the patient suddenly developed an idiosyncrasy to the drug, not unlike anaphylaxis.[17] A singular case of fatal secondary toxic thrombocytopenic purpura was ascribed to sensitization to sodium salicylate.[39]

Personal Experiment

A personal experiment, undertaken some three years ago, may be interesting enough for insertion at this place. Ingestion of 12 aspirin tablets daily resulted after five days in spontaneous profuse nosebleed. In order to check on the reliability of this observation the test was repeated twice over, with precisely the same results. The proof seemed to be all the more convincing as the author had not experienced nosebleed for more than fifty years.

The mode of action of the salicylates and their effect on prothrombin levels have been widely studied, but there is still little unanimity on the subject. Smith,[44] in reviewing the evidence, arrived at the following conclusion: "The salicylates are among the least toxic of commonly used drugs; but rarely, even in moderate doses, they produce severe reactions, particularly in asthmatic patients. Large doses may produce a transient fall in plasma prothrombin, but there is seldom a hemorrhagic tendency." Earlier, Quick[37] had expressed doubt whether salicylates could decrease the prothrombin of the blood to such a degree as to cause hemorrhage, and cautioned that the possibility should not be ignored that salicylates might cause hemorrhage in ways other than through prothrombin. Fashena and Walker[13] found in every one of their cases marked prolongation of prothrombin time, 24 hours after start of administration of salicylates. Hypoprothrombinemia reached a maximum by the second day, declining thereafter despite continued salicylate therapy. These findings were questioned by others,[16] and doubt was expressed whether the small doses of salicylates commonly used in the practice of medicine could produce hypoprothrombinemia.[6]

The evidence as to the relation of amount of ingested salicylate or blood salicylate level, and the severity of hypoprothrombinemia is also controversial. The plasma salicylate level in a given individual cannot be predicted from the dose administered.[5] Furthermore, an increased dosage of salicylate does not seem to result in an added increase in the prothrombin time, after elevation has once been produced.[4] Other observers found no effect on prothrombin values even with a blood salicylate level of approximately 35 mg.[7]

In spite of all this the prothrombinopenic effect of salicylic acid cannot be doubted. The salicylates have a similar molecular structure as dicumarol,[5] of which salicylic acid is a degradation product.[27 41] However, salicylic acid is only about one-twentieth as potent in its prothrombinopenic action as dicumarol.[19 21] This similarity is drastically demonstrated in a detailed case report by Rice, Ackerman and Saichek.[40]

A patient was kept for a total of 51 months on dicumarol therapy in order to prevent recurrences of thromboembolic episodes. For this purpose prothrombin levels were maintained between 20 and 50 per cent. However, they became depressed when in addition to dicumarol, salicylates or sulfonamides were administered. The patient was himself a physician and therefore able to describe the development in detail: "The lower levels occurred only during periods when I received aspirin or sulfonamides. Dicumarol dosage has been since readjusted to avoid critically low levels during periods when these drugs are being taken. This phenomenon became apparent late in 1946 when I began to note gingival bleeding (bloody toothbrush) during a period when my usual dicumarol medication was supplemented by aspirin and sulfonamides. This sign had repeatedly occurred before its significance was realized and mirrored the low prothrombin levels, which were demonstrated at that time. Besides a bloody tooth brush, petechiae, conjunctival hemorrhages, ecchymosis of the skin, hematuria, and bloody stools also occurred. Mild gastro-intestinal disturbances seemed to precede the onset of hemorrhagic phenomena and consist of distention, flatulence, abdominal cramps, and light to clay-colored stools. These episodes have been avoided by reducing dicumarol dosage during salicylate or sulfonamide therapy."

These observations demonstrate beyond any doubt the similarity of the effect produced by aspirin, the sulfonamides, and dicumarol. Indeed, antithrombotic prophylaxis was as effectively maintained when aspirin was partly substituted for dicumarol. In this respect the case reported by Rice and his coworkers is the clinical confirmation of earlier experiments in animals: "The complementary action of salicylate and dicumarol may be important in the clinical use of the latter. Their accidental concomitant administration may be the basis for some of the extraordinary responses observed in man. Both drugs might under certain conditions be given simultaneously to advantage. Work in Link's laboratory (unpublished) indicates that animals can be kept mildly prothrombinopenic without manifestations of bleeding, by first giving a moderate dose of dicumarol followed by smaller dicumarol-salicylate dosage . . . The action of salicylate is apparently identical with that of the anticoagulant dicumarol, but less effective. The two drugs can complement each other."[42]

When seen in the context of these clinical and experimental findings, our own observations — though not arrived at under strictly scientific conditions — may be of therapeutic interest. A regular intake of aspirin is advised to all male patients in the age bracket between 45 and 65 years, and especially to those who are overweight,[2] apparently have a tendency to overeat, and lead a sedentary life with little or no physical exercise. In the beginning it was thought necessary to recommend 10 to 30 grains of acetylsalicylic acid daily,[3] but in the course of time it was found that one or two tablets (5 to 10 grains) are sufficiently effective. These individuals seem to do well even with as little as five tablets of aspirin a week, but in order to build up a regular habit the rule of 'one aspirin a day' has been adopted. During the past seven years this regimen was recommended to 1465 subjects who were seen for a number of complaints unrelated to the cardiovascular system. All returned at regular intervals, and not one of them developed coronary occlusion or coronary insufficiency. In such a large number of subjects of this type most likely to experience coronary episodes it is — to say the least—remarkable that all remained healthy and active. Such a finding is contrary to statistical expectations, as well as to the consistent experience of 36 years in general practice, and furnishes an indication as to the therapeutic value of regular intake of small doses of acetylsalicylic acid.

Effectiveness of Small Doses

The effectiveness of such small doses of aspirin in the prevention of coronary thrombosis is, of course, surprising. Yet how to explain the fact that a subject to whom the aspirin regimen was suggested, but who simply could not be bothered to carry it through, suffered an acute attack of coronary thrombosis two months later? Should all these findings simply be written off as nothing but coincidence? This same patient, after having recovered from the attack and being discharged by the cardiologist who had attended him during his illness, was started with permission of the latter on the prophylactic aspirin regimen, and has now remained without recurrences for two years.

During the past three years 18 additional patients took to the simple aspirin formula after recuperating from their first coronary attack, and all of them have remained well and without recurrences of cardiovascular episodes. In some cases patients had been condemned to a life of semi-invalidism, but have now returned to a normal active routine. Attending cardiologists agreed that such a small amount of aspirin could do no harm, and were willing to give the procedure a fair trial. Patients who kept to the aspirin regimen and at the same time cut down a little on the size of their meals felt the effect progressively, and in the course of a few months were able to mow lawns, do gardening, and other work as before the coronary attack.

This series of observations is much too small to warrant any definite claims concerning the effectiveness of low-dosage acetylsalicylic acid therapy for the prevention of coronary thrombosis. Only a large number of cases, initially examined as to cardiovascular status, and carefully followed up over a number of years could substantiate the value of the described procedure. As long as the effectiveness of aspirin in the prophylaxis of coronary thrombosis was suspected merely on the basis of scientific demonstrations and personal observations, nothing more than a tentative course of procedure seemed to be permissible. Every possible precaution was taken to conduct these preliminary observations in a manner designed to benefit the subject without incurring any risk. Aspirin, one or two daily, was advised to all these subjects with the wish that by this simple means, they might be spared the cruel agony or untimely death due to coronary thrombosis.

Future observations bearing upon the effectiveness of the salicylates might be made by gradually substituting salicylates, and particularly aspirin for dicumarol. The case reported by Rice and his co-workers[40] definitely suggests the feasibility of such a trial in certain phases of long-term prophylactic therapy or coronary episodes.

Experimentation with the anticoagulants has been developed step by step. The sequence of events is especially clear with regard to medication with dicumarol. Starting from observations on the hemorrhagic disease of cattle, the drug was isolated from spoiled sweet clover hay, and its properties regarding coagulation and prothrombin time of blood were first demonstrated in animal experiments, and later in humans. Even though the primarily prophylactic quality of the anticoagulants[24] was soon recognized, dicumarol was initially employed merely to forestall exacerbating complications of acute thrombotic conditions, particularly in postoperative thrombophlebitis. With gratifying successes the field of application was gradually extended to include similar conditions, and among them acute coronary occlusion with myocardial infarction.[47] Again medication started with the prevention of complications of acute episodes, and only later the therapy was cautiously extended to include long-term medication for the prevention of repeated coronary attacks. Thus experimental and clinical research followed a logical plan, carefully exploring new possibilities of anticoagulant therapy.

Will experimental and clinical research in its slow but steady progress eventually test the observations here presented? Only the future can tell whether they are finally to be substantiated or refuted. The achievements of anticoagulant therapy during the last decade are almost incredible, and have resulted in preservation of lives in cases which would formerly have been considered beyond human help.[14,47] Thus the day may not be too distant when anticoagulant therapy will be extended to the period **before** the first coronary attack, starting with those cases in which definite premonitory signs can be detected.

The effectiveness of very small doses of aspirin, never exceeding 30 grains (2 gram) daily, but mostly amounting to only 5 grains (⅓ grams) daily, is in itself surprising. Lowering of the prothrombin level had ordinarily been observed only after administration of much larger doses. But it must be taken into consideration that experimental and clinical study of the action of the salicylates was mainly undertaken to test the toxicity of the drug in amounts desirable for antirheumatic therapy. However, there are cases on record, for instance case No. 1 in the report of Zimmerman and Shapiro,[48] in which a dose of 2 grams of aspirin resulted in a significant increase of prothrombin time. Meyer and Howard[27] reported consistent significant increase of prothrombin time and coagulation time following administration of 20 grains (1.3 grams) to normal individuals.

Another point requiring further investigation is the finding that the prothrombinopenic effect of salicylates often declines after a period of days or weeks, and readings return to about normal, despite the maintenance of high levels of salicylate concentration in the blood.[34] If our observations are correct, aspirin acts as an anticoagulant over months or years. Could it be that minimum doses possess a different action pattern as compared with massive amounts of salicylates? Particularly, could it be that the initial response toward small doses persists over long periods of time while larger amounts tend to create a tolerance for the drug? Furthermore, even a marginal reduction of blood coagulability might have an as yet unknown effect upon other factors responsible for the development of coronary thrombosis, tipping, as it were, the balance in favor of the patient. These are points to be considered in future specific experiments and clinical research.

All the unsolved problems connected with the observations here presented should, however, not deter from testing aspirin medication for the nonspecific prevention of coronary thrombosis. The amount of salicylate administered is so small that no side effects have to be expected, even from prolonged administration of the drug. The therapy is inexpensive, easily supervised, and will hardly ever interfere with other procedures which might become necessary. Thus the least that can be said is that it will not be injurious, and we feel that it is up to the general practitioner to give aspirin therapy for the prevention of coronary thrombosis a fair trial.

Summary

Aspirin (acetylsalicylic acid), taken consistently in small daily doses, has proved valuable in the nonspecific prophylaxis of coronary thrombosis, before the first attack, as well as in the prevention of recurrences. The series is too small to be statistically significant, and observations were not carried out under scientific conditions. However, the anticoagulative properties of aspirin cannot be doubted, and others have reported earlier that acetylsalicylic acid is a valuable adjunct to dicumarol in long-term anticoagulative therapy. The observations presented will have to be confirmed by clinical research. But they suggest strongly that aspirin medication for nonspecific prophylaxis of coronary thrombosis is an inexpensive and innocuous procedure whose possible benefits should not be overlooked by the general practitioner.

References

1. Ashworth, C. T., and McKemie, J. F.: Hemorrhagic complications, with death probably from salicylate therapy. J.A.M.A. **126:** 806-810, Nov. 25, 1944.
2. Baker, T. W., and Willius, F. A.: Coronary thrombosis among women. Am. J. Med. Sc. **196:** 315-818, Dec. 1938.
3. Binz, C.: Vorlesungen Ueber Pharmakologie, Berlin, 2nd ed., 1891.
4. Butt, H. R., Leake, W. H., Solley, R. F., Griffith, G. C., Huntington, R. W., and Montgomery, H.: Studies in rheumatic fever. I. The physiologic effect of sodium salicylate on the human being, with particular reference to the prothrombin level of the blood and the effect on hepatic parenchyma. J.A.M.A. **128:** 1195-1200, Aug. 25, 1945.
5. Clausen, F. W., and Jager, B. V.: The relation of the plasma salicylate level to the degree of hypoprothrombinemia. J. Lab. & Clin. Med. **31:** 428-436, April 1946.
6. Coombs, F. S., Higley, C. S., and Warren, H. A.: The magnitude of salicylate hypoprothrombinemia. Proc. Am. Fed. Clin. Res. **2:** 57-58, 1945.
7. Coombs, F. S., Warren, H. A., and Higley, C. S.: Toxicity of salicylates. J. Lab. & Clin. Med. **30:** 378-379, April 1945.
8. Craven, L. L.: Acetylsalicylic acid, possible preventive of coronary thrombosis. Ann. West. Med. & Surg. **4:** 95-99, Feb. 1950.
9. Dale, D. U., and Jaques, L. B.: The prevention of experimental thrombosis by dicumarin. Canad. M.A.J **46:** 546-548, June 1942.
10. Doles, H. M.: Prothrombin determinations in acute coronary occlusions. South. Med. J. **36:** 709-713, Nov. 1943.
11. Editorial: Acetylsalicylic acid deaths. J.A.M.A. **115:** 1199, Oct. 5, 1940.
12. Ersner, M. S., Myers, D., and Ersner, W.: A clinical and experimental study of the action of saliva on blood coagulation and wound healing in surgery of the oral cavity and throat. Ann. Otol. Rhin. & Laryng. **43:** 114-115, March 1934.
13. Fashena, G. J., and Walker, J. N.: Salicylate intoxication. Studies on the effects of sodium salicylate on prothrombin time and alkali reserve. Am. J. Dis. Child. **68:** 369-375, Dec. 1944.

14. Felder, D. A.: Evaluation of the various clinical signs of thrombophlebitis and experience in therapy with anticoagulants. Surg. Gynec. & Obst. 88: 337-350. March 1949.

15. Foley, W. T., and Wright, I. S.: Long-term anticoagulant therapy for cardiovascular diseases. Am. J. Med. Sc. 217: 136-142, Feb. 1949

16. Govan, C. D., Jr.: The effect of salicylate administration on the prothrombin time. J. Pediat. 29: 629-636, Nov. 1946.

17. Heindl, I. A., Anderson, B. G., and Friedlander, R. D.: Acute idiopathic hypoprothrombinemia, response to massive doses of vitamin K. Ann. Int. Med. 29: 347-356. Aug. 1948.

18. Hilton, J. H. B., Cameron, W. M., Mills, E. S., and Townsend, S. R.: The questionable importance of blood changes in coronary occlusion. Canad. M.A.J. 59: 447-452, Nov. 1948.

19. Jaques, L. B., and Lepp, E.: Action of sodium salicylate on prothrombin time in rabbits. Proc. Soc. Exper. Biol. & Med. 66: 178-181, Oct. 1947.

20. Konzelmann, F. W.: Pathologic aspects of blood coagulation. Ann. West. Med. & Surg. 4: 66-68, Feb. 1950.

21. Link, K. P.: The anticoagulant 3.3' methylenebis (4-hydroxycoumarin). Fed. Proc. 4: 176-182, June 1945.

22. Link, K. P., Overman, R. S., Sullivan, W. R., Huebner, C. F., and Scheel, L. D.: Studies on the hemorrhagic sweet clover disease. XI. Hypoprothrombinemia in the rat induced by salicylic acid. J. Biol. Chem. 147: 463-474, Feb. 1943.

23. Loewe, L., Hirsch, E., Grayzel, D. M., and Kashdan, F.: Experimental study of the comparative action of heparin and dicumarol on the in vivo clot. J. Lab. & Clin. Med. 33: 721-732. June 1948.

24. Marple, Charles D., and Wright, Irving S.: Thromboembolic Conditions and Their Treatment with Anticoagulants. Springfield, Ill., Charles C. Thomas, 1950, p. 63.

25. Marple, Charles D., and Wright, Irving S.: Thromboembolic Conditions and Their Treatment with Anticoagulants. Springfield, Ill., Charles C. Thomas, 1950, p. 271.

26. Master, A. M., and Jaffe, H. L.: Factors in the onset of coronary occlusion and coronay insufficiency. J. A. M. A. 148: 794-798, March 8, 1952.

27. Meyer, O. O., and Howard, B.: Production of hypoprothrombinemia and hypocoagulability of the blood with salicylates. Proc. Soc. Exper. Biol. & Med. 53: 234-237, June 1943.

28. Meyers, L., and Poindexter, C. A.: A study of the prothrombin time in normal subjects and in patients with arteriosclerosis. Am. Heart J. 31: 27-32, Jan. 1946.

29. Modell, W., and Patterson, R.: Intestinal bleeding associated with acetylsalicylic acid. J.A.M.A. 147: 124-126, Sept. 8, 1951.

30. Neivert, H.: Late secondary tonsillar hemorrhage. Arch. Otolaryng. 42: 14-18, July 1945.

31. Nicol, E. S.: The risk of hemorrhage in anticoagulant therapy. Ann. West. Med. & Surg. 4: 71-81, Feb. 1950.

32. Nichol, E. S., and Fassett, D. W.: An attempt to forestall acute coronary thrombosis. South. Med. J. 40: 631-637, Aug. 1947.

33. Ogura, J. H., Fetter, N. R., Blankenhorn, M. A., and Glueck, H. I.: Changes in blood coagulation following coronary thrombosis measured by the heparin retared clotting test (Waugh and Ruddick test). J. Clin. Invest. 25: 586-596, July 1946.

34. Owen, G. C., and Bradford, H. A.: The prothrombinopenic effect of massive salicylate therapy in acute rheumatic fever. Ann. Int. Med. 25: 97-102, July 1946.

35. Plotz, M.: The preventive aspects of coronary disease and myocardial infarction. New York State J. Med. 44: 1227-1229, June 1, 1944.

36. Quick, A. J.: The anticoagulants effective in vivo with special reference to heparin and dicumarol. Physiol. Rev. 24: 297-318, July, 1944.

37. Quick, A. J.: Salicylates and hemorrhage. J.A.M.A. 126: 1167, Dec. 30, 1944.

38. Rapoport, S., Wing, M., and Guest, G. M.: Hypoprothrombinemia after salicylate arministration in man and rabbits. Proc. Soc. Exper. Biol. & Med. 53: 40-41, May 1943.

39. Rappoport, A. E., Nixon, C. E., and Barker, W. A.: Fatal secondary, toxic thrombocytopenic purpura due to sodium salicylate. J. Lab. & Clin. Med. 30: 916-927, Nov. 1945.

40. Rice, R. L., Ackerman, J. S., and Saichek, R.: Long-term dicumarol therapy. Ann. Int. Med. 32: 735-745, April 1950.

41. Shapiro, S.: Studies on prothrombin. VI. The effect of synthetic vitamin K on the prothrombinopenia induced by salicylate in man. J.A.M.A. 125: 546-548, June 24, 1944.

42. Shapiro, S., Redish, M. H., and Campbell, H. A.: Studies on prothrombin. IV. The prothrombinopenic effect of salicylate in man. Proc. Soc. Exper. Biol. & Med. 53: 251-254, June 1943.

43. Singer, R.: Acetylsalicylic acid, a probable cause for secondary post-tonsillectomy hemorrhage. Arch. Otolaryng. 42: 19-20, July 1945.

44. Smith, P. K.: Certain aspects of the pharmacology of the salicylates. Pharmacol. Rev. (J. Pharmacol. & Exper. Therap., Part 2) 1: 353-382, Dec. 1949.

45. Stevens, D. L., and Kaplan, D. B.: Salicylate intoxication in children. Am. J. Dis. Child. 70: 331-335, Nov.-Dec. 1945.

46. Wintrobe, Maxwell M.: Clinical Hematology, 3rd ed. Philadelphia, Lea & Febiger, 1951, p. 967

47. Wright, I. S.: The use of the anticoagulants in the treatment of diseases of the heart and blood vessels. Ann. Int. Med. 30: 80-91, Jan. 1949.

48. Zimmerman, S. P., and Shapiro, S.: Correlation between salicylate dosage and plasma level and the prothrombin content of the blood. Exper. Med. & Surg. 4: 110-117, May 1946.

A single inspiring quotation or article may change the entire course of your life—may give it new purpose and direction, new meaning, new hope.

Appendix 3

An edited and annotated extract from the Witness Seminar, 'Thrombolysis', 28 January 2003[227]

Streptokinase Trials (1986–96)

Professor Brian Pentecost (Chair): One tends to think of the development of thrombolysis in clinical practice, as dating back to the late 1980s, when the big studies – the International Study of Infarct Survival (ISIS), Gruppo Italiano per lo Studio della Streptochinasi nell'Infarto Miocardico (GISSI) and Global Utilization of Streptokinase and tPA [tissue plasminogen activator] for Occluded Coronary Arteries (GUSTO) – were published.[228] But in fact streptokinase had been around for a very long time. I looked at its history with the licensing authority. It was being used intermittently in varying doses, for various conditions before drugs were licensed in the UK. In 1973 it was issued with a Licence of Right, which was simply an acknowledgement that it had been in use and it didn't imply efficacy. It was nearly 20 years on, in 1991, when it was given a full licence after review.[229] The studies I have mentioned played a large part in obtaining that full licence. The drug, of course, was *Streptase* by Hoeschst.

Professor Desmond Julian: The first presentation on the subject of streptokinase and myocardial infarction (MI) was by Fletcher and Sherry in 1957.[230] Their paper was published in 1959. Some people were quite quick off the mark, including Dr Dewar, and I am very happy to see him in the audience, because in 1961 along with two other groups, he published a pilot

---

[227] The unpublished transcript of this Witness Seminar will be deposited in Archives and Manuscripts, Wellcome Library, London, along with other records of the meeting.

[228] ISIS (1987); GISSI (1986); GUSTO (1993).

[229] Product Licences of Right were granted in the early 1970s for the brand names *Kabinkinase* (Kabivitrum) and *Streptase* (Hoechst). The Medicines Control Agency granted full reviewed marketing authorization to *Kabinkinase* in 1989 and to *Streptase* in 1991, as published in the London, Edinburgh and Belfast Gazette [freely available at www.gazettes-online.co.uk/ (visited 4 May 2005)]. E-mail from Mark Goddard of the Medicines and Healthcare Products Regulatory Agency to Mrs Lois Reynolds, 8 April 2005.

[230] Fletcher *et al.* (1959a and b).

study on the use of streptokinase in myocardial infarction and then he expanded the series. Please correct me if I have got this wrong, Hewan. He expanded the series a couple of years later into a study of 75 patients.[231] Unfortunately, perhaps because the study was small, or perhaps using the wrong preparation, that was not positive. And over the succeeding years there are quite a large number of studies, some randomized, some mis-randomized, and some truly randomized. In 1967 we held what happened to be the first conference on Coronary Care in Edinburgh. At that meeting Chazov,[232] whose name you may know having won the Nobel Peace Prize, who at that time was the cardiologist to the Kremlin and all the leaders of the Soviet Union and on the Politbureau, told us that streptokinase was widely used in the Soviet Union in 1967, that it made the electrocardiogram (ECG) evolve more quickly, the infarct healed more quickly, and all sorts of things which were rediscovered ten or 15 years later by everybody else. But it was widely used in the Soviet Union at that time.[233]

Then there were a number of major studies in the succeeding years. There was one in 1971, which showed a significant benefit.[234] There was a European cooperative study in 1979, which I think raised eyebrows because the mortality in the control group was 30 per cent and the mortality in the streptokinase group was 15 per cent.[235] We found that very difficult to believe, and we thought these patients were not being very well looked after. Actually they had excluded low-risk cases, so I think it's probably not quite as bad a reflection on management at that time as it might appear. And then in the late 1980s, GISSI and the Second International Study of Infarct Survival (ISIS-2) came along.

I am very pleased to see Sir Richard Doll in the audience, because he can correct me. Doll was the leader of the data monitoring committee, I have forgotten what we called it then, Sir Richard, but whatever it was. You all

---

[231] Dewar *et al.* (1961, 1963).

[232] The Nobel Peace Prize for 1985 was awarded to the cofounders of the International Physicians for the Prevention of Nuclear War, Professor Bernard Lown from the USA and Professor Yevgeny Chazov from the Soviet Union, a Moscow cardiologist and Soviet Deputy Minister of Health.

[233] Chazov (1965). For a later overview, see Rapaport (1991).

[234] Dioguardi *et al.* (1971).

[235] European Cooperative Study Group for Streptokinase Treatment in Acute Myocardial Infarction (1979).

know, of course, the results of GISSI and ISIS-2, but we were faced with a particular problem during the conduct of the trial, when in the first 4000 patients treated under four hours,[236] there was a very, very highly significant reduction in mortality.[237] The decision was taken to publish a letter in the *Lancet* to inform people of this result, and suggest that it was up to the individual physician to decide whether they should continue that therapy in that subgroup of patients or not. As it happened, Sir Richard, you can correct me, but I think most physicians continued to prescribe, at least to enter patients into the trial, and as a consequence there were quite a lot of patients who died not having received streptokinase, who might not have died had they done so. I must say I feel rather uncomfortable about the decision and I would be very interested to know what Sir Richard feels about that. But I think once we reached that publication in 1988 the situation was quite clear, that the role of thrombolysis had been clearly established.[238]

One other issue and that is the use of intracoronary streptokinase, because Dr Dewar here perhaps was the pioneer in doing this on seven cases, I think, and Roger Smith, who's sitting there, did the work of pushing the streptokinase into the coronary arteries. Rentrop[239] gained a great deal of reputation later on, and indeed an international reputation for doing the same thing eventually in a large number of patients. Of course, intracoronary streptokinase was eventually found to be no better perhaps than intravenous streptokinase, but it's an interesting chapter in the history of thrombolysis.

Dr Arthur Hollman: I think Bill Fulton – Fulton and Sumner in fact – made an immense contribution to the understanding of coronary thrombosis while working in Glasgow in 1976, perhaps surprisingly late in a way. We have heard that Dr Hewan Dewar was working in 1961, and Fulton and Sumner published in 1976 in the *British Heart Journal*.[240] But for those who don't know the work, very briefly, they did what I think was really a rather remarkable thing. Everybody who came into their hospital in Glasgow with an acute

---

[236] Professor Julian said later in the meeting: 'I was wrong, it was six hours and not four.' See page 100.

[237] GISSI (1986, 1987); Franzosi *et al.* (1987); ISIS (1987).

[238] ISIS-2 (1988).

[239] Hugenholtz and Rentrop (1982). Rentrop *et al.* (1980). See also Merx *et al.* (1981).

[240] Fulton and Sumner (1976).

myocardial infarction had an injection of radiolabelled fibrinogen.[241] I am not sure that would get past the ethical committees these days, but that's what was done. Maybe it was explained to them [the patients]. And then the thrombus in the coronary artery related to in the infarct of those who died was examined to see which bits of it, if any, were radioactive. If the thrombus has been the result of the infarction, then the whole of the thrombus would have been radioactive, because the fibrinogen was given beforehand. In fact, they found the reverse, they found that the thrombus related to the infarct was radionegative, so that indicated very clearly indeed it was a thrombus that gave rise to the infarct and not vice versa.

Dr Hewan Dewar: The first thing that I did was a pilot study of intravenous streptokinase in 1961 and a full one in 1963.[242] As Desmond has hinted, there were defects in this study and I think it's worth considering whether the publication did more harm than good. There were quite a large number of patients when we did the proper study – 75 of them – well divided between the two groups of treated and controls, and we went to a lot of trouble to study their progress by electrocardiograms, transaminase studies, and so on, and there was really no difference.

There were one or two defects. One was the fact that we really hadn't appreciated how important it was to get patients treated early, and we thought in those days that we did quite well if treatment started up to about 12 hours, and the median was about six hours, so that really wasn't very good. The other defect that Desmond hinted at was that we actually used something that the firm said was plasminogen activated by streptokinase, and I think most people thought there was an awful lot of streptokinase in it, whereas most of it was plasmin.[243] We hadn't at that time realized how unsuitable plasmin is for systemic injection. It's extremely good for local injections into arteries, but it's very unsatisfactory for systemic use, because it becomes so diluted and then

---

[241] Dr Arthur Hollman wrote: 'He gave radiolabelled fibrinogen to patients admitted with chest pain and in those who developed an acute infarction and died, he used autoradiography to examine the thrombus in the infracted territory. The proximal thrombus – which pre-dated hospital admission – was radionegative, while the distal thrombus was radiopositive, showing it had continued to propagate after admission. His study showed beyond doubt that the thrombus came first.' Note on draft transcript, 25 March 2005.

[242] Dewar *et al.* (1961, 1963).

[243] Thrombolysin was supplied by Merck, Sharp and Dohme for both studies. See note 248.

comes against antiplasmin. For these reasons, the study produced a negative result. It was worse than that in one sense, because when I presented it somewhere I was congratulated on the design, they thought it was really an excellent way of presenting a negative result, and yet I think it probably held back the use of streptokinase for many years.

One of the rather interesting things is that just a few years after this, in 1966, a number of German and Swiss doctors published a study in which they had done very much the same thing, not quite so carefully, because their randomization wasn't so marvellous, but they had done quite a large number, some of them with what today you would call a pain-to-needle time of three-and-a-half hours, which was really, I think, absolutely wonderful.[244] But, of course, nobody had ever bothered with it, as it was published in a German periodical, and as far as I know has never seen the light of day or been quoted since. But then what it is that enables something to be quoted I think has already been well described in the *Lancet.* For an article published before 1966 to be quoted, it might just as well have been published before 1066.[245] I think if somebody had really persevered in the study of streptokinase after the publication of our negative result, and had paid attention to the German and Swiss study, then we could have had these treatments available earlier and it's a great tragedy. I can't help wondering if a negative trial isn't sometimes a disaster, even if it's quite well devised. But I would be interested to know what the rest of you think about that.

Our intravenous study had begun in 1961, and I did a variety of things between those years in the fibrinolysis sphere and was also very interested in coronary ambulances. I enlisted the help of Roger Smith, who had acquired the expertise of catheterizing coronary arteries while working in Edinburgh. The two of us, plus a very good radiologist, treated eight early cases of acute MI in 1976 by direct catheter injection of streptokinase and in 1977 showed the results to a joint autumn meeting of the British and Swedish Cardiac Societies. We had successfully lysed thrombi in three out of six, two having shown only coronary stenosis, that is a 50 per cent success rate. They were only temporary successes, because we did not give heparin at the same time for

[244] Poliwoda *et al.* (1966).

[245] The online version of PubMed, one of the databases run by the National Centre for Biotechnology Information at the US National Library of Medicine and the National Institutes of Health, established in 1988, has been available from 1950 to 2005 since 5 October 2004.

fear that the sites of catheter entry in the femoral arteries would bleed uncontrollably. In their cases, the Russians did follow with heparin. Our cases therefore did mostly clot up again, but at least they did demonstrate some clearing of the previously blocked coronary artery. They are shown in the book that Desmond [Julian] has very loyally brought with him today.[246]

The effect of our demonstration to the Cardiac Societies wasn't a bit electric, it felt like a damp squib. Only two questions were asked: one person asked me whether I had got the permission of the ethical committee, of which I am glad to say the answer was yes. The other was a much more doubting chap from Glasgow who asked me, quite sensibly, what I hoped to achieve by it. I didn't like to tell him that I hoped to shake the British Cardiac Society a bit and perhaps make some go into the whole subject of fibrinolysis in more detail. I don't remember quite what answer I gave him. I had difficulty in publishing it, because in the end the *British Medical Journal* thought it was too specialized, and the American College of Cardiology thought it wasn't really important enough and advised me to show it somewhere else. I had already given a demonstration on it to a meeting of fibrinolysis experts in Czechoslovakia, and they asked me for a text, so I gave them the article and that's where it now is, in the proceedings of that conference.[247]

I knew that the Russians were interested. There was this chap, Chazov, who had been a cardiologist in Stalin's reign, so he was evidently a man of courage. By the time I had dealings with him Stalin had died and perhaps the succeeding era required even more courage. I corresponded with him, because he had done two cases (originally I thought it was only one) of intracoronary injection of a fibrinolytic agent, with one success.[248] He had used something that he called fibrinolysin, and I finally found out what this was. It was human plasmin, derived from placentas that had been activated with trypsin and of course it might have just as well been plasmin from any source, and he had one success out of these two. I did ask him some questions, and he replied, giving me some details as to why he had used this particular preparation. He was anxious not to have to use streptokinase, because there might be antibodies in

---

[246] Dewar (1998): 53.

[247] Dewar (1979). Papers presented at the Fourth International Conference on Synthetic Fibrinolytic Thrombolytic Agents and at the Fourth Pilzen Symposium on Thrombosis held at Karlovy Vary and Pilzen, Czechoslovakia, 5–8 September 1978.

[248] Chazov *et al.* (1977).

the blood stream, which was perhaps a fair comment. But in the last bit of his letter to me, which did surprise me, he said that he thought that this method of treatment had a long-range future. Coming from a cardiologist at the centre of Russia, you may wonder what was meant by long-range usefulness of intracoronary fibrinolysis for coronary thrombosis.

Pentecost: Actually you do have a publication in the *British Heart Journal*, in the *Proceedings*, it's the autumn meeting of 1977. It's where these beautiful pictures were shown.[249]

Dewar: Yes, but the full description is in this rather forgotten *Proceedings* of the Fibrinolysis Society, whose total title I have forgotten.

Sir Richard Doll: I had some ethical difficulty in taking on the chairmanship of the Data Monitoring Committee (DMC) of this trial, because I was quite convinced that both aspirin and streptokinase were useful and in fact I made it a condition of being Chairman of the DMC that if I had a MI during the course of the trial I was to have aspirin and streptokinase. So that put me in a slightly difficult position. But I have always thought that ethical considerations of an individual physician and of a DMC for a big trial are different. The clinician to my mind, as soon as he has any gut feeling that one treatment probably is better than the other, he will probably want to give it to the next patient, and he may well do that when there are statistical differences significant only at the 5 per cent level in favour of a particular treatment in a trial. For the ISIS trial, the situation seemed to me quite different. I think other people on the committee also agreed with me that the evidence was already pretty clear, and of course the evidence was made available to all the clinicians that admitted patients to the trial, they had the results of the meta-analysis which Collins and Peto had carried out, which showed the beneficial effects.[250] But there were occasional cases of cerebral haemorrhage and this apparently put off a lot of cardiologists, certainly in Sweden. I know that from a discussion with Lars Wilhelmsen. The Swedes were very concerned with the possibility of cerebral haemorrhage. They were not admitting patients to the trial. Well our view on the DMC was that we would report the results, we weren't responsible for continuing the trial or stopping it, but we would report the results to the management committee, when in our view the results were such as to be likely

---

[249] Dewar *et al.* (1978).

[250] Yusuf *et al.* (1985).

to change medical practice. There's no point in doing these big trials unless the results are going to be taken notice of, and we therefore said we will report the results when in our view they are such as will change medical practice. Eventually we confidently reported to the management committee that treatment, I think under six hours, was very clearly beneficial. To our astonishment, the management committee didn't pay any attention to that. Or rather they paid some attention, but they didn't stop the trial. What they did was to inform people of the results that we reported, and the result of it was that actually a higher number of patients were admitted, particularly in Sweden, where they had been so frightened of the risk of haemorrhage, and the trial was continued. Our view of the evidence that it would change medical practice turned out to be wrong. It still wasn't strong enough to do so.

If I may just add one side comment? The other drug that was being used in that ISIS-2 trial was aspirin and the DMC were seriously criticized for not having stopped the trial earlier because the benefits of aspirin were so clear. The interesting thing is that at the time the final report was made to the management committee when they did stop the trial, the data in the hands of the DMC showed only marginal benefit from aspirin, and it was just the results that came in after we had reported to the management committee that swung the results in favour of aspirin to such an extent that people asked, not unreasonably, 'Why the hell did you go on and allow treatment without aspirin to be carried on for so long?' I think those are the points I wanted to make and they do, I think, raise some quite important issues in relation to what the function of the data monitoring committee is and I wanted to put them before you.

Julian: First, I was wrong, it was six hours and not four.[251] Yes, I remember the aspirin business very clearly, because this is, I think, quite an interesting point for a data monitoring committee. We actually looked at data of hospital discharge, because a lot of the benefit was in the remaining period between discharge and 35 days. So when they told us the results I was personally very surprised that it was as positive as it was.

Pentecost: We will come to the large trials that we have been mentioning a little later, but are there some more comments on the very early periods of thrombolysis, pre-ISIS-2?

---

[251] See note 236.

Professor John Hampton: I remember going to a meeting in Phoenix, Arizona, in 1969, when this was discussed, and as I remember it there were two things discussed there. One was a belief that thrombosis was something to do with platelets and fibrinolysis was something to do with clotting and therefore probably wouldn't work. The other thing was a really marked worry about bleeding. And it was the fear of bleeding that really put people off using thrombolysis on the basis of the sort of evidence we have heard so far.

Pentecost: There was a very good review paper published in 1985 by Yusuf, Peto and Collins in the *European Heart Journal*.[252] They identified about 6000 patients with myocardial infarct (MI) who had been randomized to treatment with streptokinase, but they pointed out that the dose regimes were extremely variable. The usual regime – I think it may have been so in your study, Hewan – was 250 000 units over 30 minutes, that's one-sixth of the dose used in the major studies that we are coming to in a moment. [**Dewar**: I think it was 500 000 over about ten hours]. But the point is that it would not have been possible in the mid-1980s, I think, to advocate routine use, because there simply wasn't a dose regime worked out. The other big problem was, as John and Sir Richard have referred to, the fear of bleeding. Has anybody else anything to contribute to this early story?

Doll: John Honour was doing the experimental work and he certainly demonstrated an effect,[253] but I think the demonstration of an effect on platelets presumably *in vitro* had been done a lot earlier and was what made most people want to use it. But people were not using aspirin and the first, what we now call meta-analysis, I don't like the term, that was done in this country in the modern efficient way was done by Richard Peto, but he published it in an unsigned editorial in the *British Medical Journal*, so people don't know that it was his work. He analysed six studies of aspirin.[254] And of course, the last, the biggest one, the American study, had not shown a positive result, and people all believed this last big study and not the six studies which when taken together clearly showed a benefit, as Elwood and Cochrane had originally shown that it would. But it was the meta-analysis of these six studies that convinced us of its benefit. But when I spoke to the Cardiological Society before we started our randomized study of the possibility of preventing MI by

---

[252] Yusuf *et al.* (1985b).

[253] Emmons *et al.* (1965). See also note 255.

[254] Anonymous (1980).

people taking aspirin prophylactically, how many were using aspirin in the treatment of myocardial infarction? The answer was 5 per cent. But following ISIS-2 it changed to 95 per cent within a matter of months, but it was 5 per cent before.

Hampton: If I could just comment on Arthur's question and Sir Richard's memory of John Honour's work, which was done before Sir Richard took the department over – it was done in George Pickering's time.[255] What they were mainly interested in when I joined the department was *Persantin®* (dipyridamole), which of course is now much more widely used. But it was the rabbit ears' model that really demonstrated that dipyridamole had an effect.[256] I don't remember them ever testing aspirin on that model.

Pentecost: I wonder too if there wasn't a rather negative view of treatments for MI in the 1970s, after the introduction of the defibrillators led to coronary care units. There were a lot of false dawns – prophylactic use of anti-arrhythmics, glucose, potassium, insulin and others. There was a sceptical attitude around, which might have made it a little more difficult to enthuse over thrombolysis. Desmond, do you think that's possible?

Julian: You are quite right. I think it is true that there was some scepticism. In fact, the concentration in the 1970s was entirely on arrhythmias, probably inappropriately. But as we pointed out, I think what the issues were, the variability of dose, the very varying results in the different trials, Hewan's already referred to them, quite a number of negative trials; the rather dubious character of the trials in terms of randomization. I think the quality of the

---

[255] Professor John Hampton wrote: 'John Honour was technician to Sir Thomas Lewis and then to George Pickering at St Mary's Hospital Medical School, London, and moved with Pickering to Oxford to be chief technician. As well as running the lab he had his own research projects, and when I joined the department in 1965 he was working with Tony Mitchell on thrombosis. Between them they had devised the "rabbit head" model which involved removing a disc of skull and exposing the arteries on the brain cortex. Under a dissecting microscope an artery was squeezed with very fine forceps, and at the injury site a "white body" would form. This was shown to be a platelet mass. These bodies would embolize repeatedly, and reform at the injured site. The frequency of embolization could be timed and used as an endpoint to study the effect of anti-platelet agents. The most important thing they discovered was that dipyridamole (*Persantin®*) was, in this model, a powerful anti-thrombotic. It was much less effective in preventing the aggregation of human platelets, and this led to a lot of interest in the differences between models of thrombosis and the differences between species.' E-mail to Mrs Lois Reynolds, 27 April 2005.

[256] Honour and Mitchell (1964).

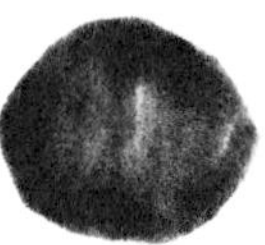

research, generally speaking, was not of a high order, the risk of bleeding was considered to be substantial. There was the question of whether thrombosis had anything to do with it. So a whole range of reasons why there was scepticism I think.

Doll: May I just add, of course, that John Hampton is correct. I apologize, John Honour's experimental work was on *Persantin*®, not on aspirin.[257]

Hampton: The other thing was of course that the world got totally hooked on the β-blockers, did it not? And therefore lost any interest there might have been in coronary care units and thrombolysis and what have you. I think it's a good example of fashions in medicine, that the fashion became β-blockers.[258]

Pentecost: Do you mean β-blockers in the acute stage?

Julian: Yes, and that's very interesting and actually you will remember only too well. It happened to me in Phoenix too, what they were concerned about was infarct size limitation and they were talking about β-blockers and calcium antagonists and so forth, whereas the important thing about infarct size is thrombolysis.

Pentecost: A lot of that followed the Sobell work didn't it? I mean the experimental work?

Julian: In fact none of it worked.

Dr Roger Smith: Yes, I was there and for the record I would like to say that it was one of the most horrific moments in my life when my boss, Dr Dewar, said that we would take the next patient with a myocardial infarction to the cath lab and stick a coronary catheter down the appropriate artery and infuse it with streptokinase, and I can't describe the sweaty fear I felt through all the cases. We did do one quite interesting case. Actually it was my fault. I knocked a clot off a prosthetic aortic valve down the coronary artery and we gave that patient streptokinase and dissolved the blockage. There was indeed a frosty reception at the Cardiac Society. My second fear was that Dr Dewar, as he went off to India, gave me the spool of film and the paper to read at the Cardiac Society, and those of you old enough will remember that it wasn't the nice, kind, society it is now. Dr Dewar said he hoped to arrive back from India in time to come along to the meeting and give the paper, otherwise I would be

---

[257] See note 255.

[258] See, for example, Snow (1965); Norwegian Multicentre Study Group (1981); and reviews in Yusuf *et al.* (1985a); Freemantle *et al.* (1999).

giving it. I remember a third comment, somebody suggested that all we did was push the clot down the artery.

Dewar: It took him 25 years to confess to me that he thought at the time that I was mad.

Pentecost: Tom Quinn, you were not there at the time.

Professor Tom Quinn: No, I feel humbled really, as I was only just born when Dr Dewar's paper was published in 1961. I want to ask if you were to attempt to do some of these things today, then the regulations around informed consent for patients would make things quite difficult. What was your experience of getting the patients on board to agree to undergo what was essentially very, very experimental stuff in the early days?

Smith: Dr Dewar will have to forgive me once again. It's really quite amusing in retrospect. I remember he got the consent from the patient, certainly for the first patient I know. I remember vividly his saying to the patient: 'You are having a myocardial infarction, which is caused by a clot in your coronary artery, and we propose to unblock it.'

Dewar: There were various ways of describing our intentions. I think I was rather economical with the whole truth.

Julian: I think this point of patient consent is a very interesting one, because I talked to Professor Rutishauser who was in Zurich at the time when Grüntzig was doing his first angioplasty and he said, 'Thank God we didn't have an ethical committee in Zurich. It would never have got past.'[259]

Professor Andrew Stevens: I am much too young for this as well, but as a public health physician looking back on this now and having read up on meta-analysis and all that I am not surprised that there was no meta-analysis, I am not surprised that no one read the German literature. What surprises me is the total absence of the drug companies in all of this. If you look at the battles these days between the different preparations in thrombolysis, they are all there, loud, clear and bell-like and arguing it out in fine detail, but I am amazed that there wasn't a company pushing streptokinase at us and funding large trials at the time. Was there something very different about the world then?

---

[259] For examples of their work, see Grüntzig and Schneider (1977); Meier and Rutishauser (1985).

Pentecost: I don't think so. I believe the answer is that by the early 1970s there was a Licence of Right, there was no patent on the drug and therefore not a lot of money to be made.

Dr Robin Norris: I don't think ethics change, but our perception of them certainly does. In a trial of coronary surgery in Auckland in the early 1970s we randomized patients by the envelope method to surgery or no surgery.[260] We said to the patients that we are offering this operation to some but not all patients because we think it might help, but we didn't know. That's all we did.

I have made out a list [Table 1, page 106] of what I think are the main trials and I won't say any more about the pre-GISSI ones, except that I think that the modern history really starts with GISSI in 1986. There are two things that paved the way for that. One has been discussed – the knowledge that coronary thrombosis causes infarction, not the other way round. If one thought that the thrombus came after the infarct, then the whole rationale would change. The thrombolytic agent is something that you can give over 36 hours, and there's no great urgency. The 'time is muscle' idea has come in since GISSI. The second thing was the perception of the type 2 error, the β error, in clinical trials. Although this was known, it was not appreciated by many of us, and many trials were far too small. So GISSI was the first of the mega trials. Having said this, the trial that hasn't been mentioned that is scientifically valid is the Western Washington trial by Ward Kennedy *et al.*, in which intracoronary streptokinase was shown to reduce mortality and with only 250 patients.[261] And then GISSI (11 000 patients), and ISIS-2 (17 000), which is perhaps the most important of all the trials because it established that aspirin as well as streptokinase reduced mortality.[262] Then there was the Anistreplase Intervention Mortality Study (AIMS) trial that Desmond, I think, instigated.[263] This was a much smaller trial that was stopped early because mortality was reduced by 50 per cent. Then came the Anglo-Scandinavian Study of Early Thrombolysis (ASSET) in about 13 000 patients using alteplase.[264] These trials all showed with complete unanimity that mortality rate was reduced, as shown subsequently by meta-analysis, by about 30 per 1000

---

[260] Norris *et al.* (1981).

[261] Kennedy *et al.* (1982, 1983, 1985).

[262] See notes 237 and 238.

[263] AIMS Trial Study Group (1988).

[264] Wilcox *et al.* (1988).

Short-term fatality (about 30 days)

Thrombolysis is the most intensively studied intervention in the history of medicine. More than 200 000 patients have been enrolled in large-scale trials worldwide.[265]

Trial[266]	Drug[267]	Reference	Number of patients	Fatality(%) Control	Fatality(%) Treated
European	SK	*NEMJ* 1979; **301**:797	315	19	12
Meta-analysis	SK	*NEMJ* 1982; **307**:1180	3277	17	14
Western Washington	SK (IC)	*NEMJ* 1983; **309**:1477	250	11	4
GISSI	SK	*Lancet* 1986 **i**: 397	11,712	13	11
ISIS-2	SK+ASA	*Lancet* 1988 **ii**: 349	17,187	13	8
AIMS	Anistreplase	*Lancet* 1988 **i**: 545	1258	12	6
ASSET	Alteplase	*Lancet* 1988 **ii**: 525	7527	10	7

Long-term fatality (6 months – 10 years)

GISSI, ISIS-2, AIMS and ASSET all showed that early fatality reduction had been maintained but not increased.[268]

Left ventricular function

Trial	Drug	Reference	Number of patients	Ejection Fraction[269] Control	Ejection Fraction Treated
White	SK	*NEMJ* 1987; **317**:850	194	53 (14)%	59 (11)%
O'Rourke	Alteplase	*Circ.* 1988; **77**:1311	128	54 (12)%	61 (13)%
Simoons	SK	*JACC* 1989;**14**:1609	533	Survival at 3–7 years was related to LV function at discharge.	

Table 1: First use and development of thrombolysis on case fatality post-myocardial infarction, 1979–89.[270]
Source: Dr Robin Norris

[265] Topol (2000).

[266] For details of trials, see note 235, Stampfer *et al.* (1982), notes 261, 237, 274–7.

[267] SK = streptokinase; SK (IC) = intracoronary streptokinase; SK + ASA = streptokinase and acetylsalicylic acid (ASA or aspirin), LV function = left ventricular function.

[268] For full details of trials, see notes 272, 282, and 238.

[269] See Glossary, page 161.

[270] Table distributed at the Witness Seminar, 'Recent History of Thrombolysis', 28 January 2003.

patients treated if it was given within six hours.[271] These trials were all followed up long term, which meant in the case of GISSI, AIMS and ASSET being only six months to a year or so.[272] But ISIS-2 followed up patients for ten years. This was published in the *British Medical Journal* in 1998, and showed pretty clearly that although early fatality had been reduced, if you took the survivors of 35 days and then looked at them again after ten years, the benefit was maintained but not increased.[273]

This came as a shock to some of us, because my own involvement was with Harvey White in Auckland. I think ours was the first trial to show that intravenous as opposed to intracoronary streptokinase reduced damage to the left ventricle of survivors. We showed a 6 per cent absolute improvement in ejection fraction, 53 per cent vs 59 per cent.[274] We also looked at end-systolic volume of the left ventricle, which we had shown was a better prognostic indicator than ejection fraction, and that was reduced in treated patients as well.[275] Then Michael O'Rourke in Sydney did the same with tPA and found a 7 per cent improvement – 54 per cent in control, 61 per cent in treated patients.[276] In the long term, Martin Simoons and colleagues showed that survival at three to seven years was related to left ventricular function after treatment.[277] This, of course, is the whole basis for the 'time is muscle' adage. Thrombolytic treatment is not only saving lives, it's reducing left ventricular damage. I thought and wrote a viewpoint paper at the time arguing that you could save on numbers in trials by looking at left ventricular function as a surrogate for mortality.[278] I don't think anybody followed our suggestion, and it may be that although an improvement in ejection fraction from 53 per cent to 59 per cent, or from 54 per cent to 61 per cent in the average patient was in the right direction, the cut-off for late mortality is really lower than this. You have to get below 50 per cent ejection fraction to reduce your longevity and our results related to the flat part of the curve.

---

271 Fibrinolytic Therapy Trialists' (FTT) Collaborative Group (1994).

272 GISSI (1987); AIMS (1990); Wilcox *et al.* (1990).

273 Baigent *et al.* (1998).

274 White *et al.* (1987b). Double blind, streptokinase, propranolol, heparin.

275 White *et al.* (1987a).

276 O'Rourke *et al.* (1988).

277 Simoons *et al.* (1989).

278 Norris and White (1988).

I would just like to talk about the door-to-needle-time enthusiasm, which I think is partly misplaced, because there again it's looking at the flat part of the curve. There is a 'golden hour', and if you can give thrombolysis within the golden hour after onset of symptoms and use a fast-acting plasminogen activator, then you will save more lives. But at the time that patients are getting to hospital at two or three hours after the onset, an extra 15 minutes to half an hour probably doesn't make much difference.

Julian: I agree, although there is a benefit obviously from earlier treatment. Can I say a bit about pre-hospital treatment? If you put the pre-hospital and in-hospital trials together, it's fairly clear that gaining an hour, say, or so is valuable and it's also valuable later on. It isn't only valuable in the first hour. What was quite interesting about the pre-hospital studies was the study from Aberdeen – is John Rawles here? [No] – which had roughly 311 patients and was stopped prematurely, was published immediately in the *British Medical Journal*.[279] The study we did, the European Myocardial Infarction Project (EMIP) study of 5500 patients, which was not positive, was immediately rejected by the *Lancet*. You can speculate as to why this differential occurred. Actually it was quite funny, because I wrote to complain to the editor of the *Lancet* about this, and he wrote a charming letter back saying he would reconsider and let his better nature prevail and look at it again. Actually I was able to write back to him and say that it had been accepted for the *New England Journal of Medicine*.[280] But I think it's very clear from this that you can demonstrate in those trials the benefit of earlier treatment, which may be maximum in the first hour, but certainly is present in each of the succeeding hours up to at least six hours.

Pentecost: So we had one clear message emerging from these studies, and that was the importance of avoiding delay and of aiming for the first hour if possible. But the studies brought in uncertainty and confusion on two counts. Which was the best drug and regime? And what was the place of heparin? John, you were involved in GUSTO, what are your feelings now, looking back in a totally dispassionate and disinterested way on what has happened during that period?

Hampton: If I can just start a bit further back from that? Desmond and I were saying a little earlier on that there are fashions in medicine and the fashion of the 1980s was β blockers, calcium blockers and anti-arrhythmias, was it not? And Desmond and I argued particularly about anti-arrhythmias. ISIS used

---

[279] GREAT Group (1992); Adams *et al.* (1993).

[280] EMIP Group. (1993).

atenolol, and the acronym, of course, stood for the International Study of Infarct Survival and we in Nottingham were running a study called the TRENT study and we thought this was terribly clever because, for those of you whose geography isn't too good, the Trent is the river that runs through Nottingham. So we had ISIS versus TRENT and at that time (it's hard to believe it now) there was a sort of equal belief that either could be the winner. TRENT was the abject loser because nifedipine did absolutely nothing. Desmond was on the Data Safety and Monitoring Board (DSMB) that actually turned it off.[281] ISIS went on to ISIS-2 (the Second International Study of Infarct Survival) and there was nothing we could do with TRENT, because it was with nifedipine. We went on to ASSET [Anglo-Scandinavian Study of Early Thrombolysis].[282] I remember very well when GISSI came out, ASSET had just about started and there was an element of 'we have started so we will finish', because there was a lot of debate as to whether having one big trial which was positive with streptokinase, was it ethical at all to continue with the study of alteplase, which had only just got going. I can't quite remember how we rationalized it, but we felt I think that one study wasn't enough, and then ISIS-2 beat us to finishing. I remember Peter Sleight telling me the answer in the Oxford Union when there was a debate debate, I think, on cholesterol. Peter Sleight and I were talking at the back of the room, and he told me the results of ISIS-2. Again we were very worried as to whether we should finish off alteplase or not. By that stage, we really had pretty well finished recruiting and we decided that it should go on. I think that with this talk we have had of ethics up until now, it is interesting as to whether we should have carried on even after GISSI, because it could well be argued now that ASSET should never have been completed. If it hadn't been completed, then we would never have had a comparison of a drug other than streptokinase against placebo. One of the interesting things that came out was that alteplase did not look as if it was any better than streptokinase, and the hope was, of course, that it would be. So GUSTO got organized after that.

We then got into the phase of comparative trials and this was basically streptokinase versus something else with various sorts of heparin and what have you. It was that at this point around 1980–85 that drug company involvement became so much more important than it had been. I think up until this stage drug companies were very laid back, very hands off, saying, 'Oh that will be a good idea, why don't you do it?' Certainly with the TRENT trial the company

---

[281] Wilcox *et al.* (1986).

[282] Wilcox *et al.* (1988, 1990).

was never seen again really, once they said we could do it, they paid the bills and kept clear. But after that, particularly with alteplase, and particularly since at that point the Americans suddenly discovered clinical trials (which up to the time of GUSTO had been mainly English). From GUSTO onwards, it became American, American, American, and American, and that was really because of the market and the involvement of drug companies who were now driving clinical trials.[283] I think that all the trials that went on after that – Robin has listed some of them here [see Table 1, page 106] – the comparative studies were led by drug companies, who saw a market for their products.

We went on to do a study called INJECT where we had the prospect of seeing if streptokinase and alteplase were equivalent.[284] This was a totally new idea and we learned as we were setting it up that equivalence is in the eye of the beholder and not in the eye of the statistician, although you can wrap it up in statistical terms. And the equivalence went on and eventually it reached its *reductio ad absurdum* with COBALT (Continuous Infusion versus Double-Bolus Administration of Alteplase), which tried to show the equivalence within half a per cent and just failed to show that the two regimes were equivalent, which they really were.[285] The development from GUSTO onwards, I think, has been the reflection of the overriding importance of drug companies and that has shown itself in the next big treatment, which, of course, was ACE [angiotensin-converting enzyme] inhibitors and then statins, always drug-company led, always 'Is my drug better than somebody else's?' I think the whole philosophy changed somewhere around GUSTO from a purely academic exercise to a much more commercial exercise and all the implications that that had. That was how I saw it from that point onwards.

Norris: Just to add to what John said, a lot of these trials now show a reduction in mortality from 5 per cent to 4 per cent, and to show this needs 10 000 patients or more. In public health terms that may not be very productive.

Julian: Yes, I can correct John. AIMS actually compared anistreplase with placebo, so there was another.[286] I think one of the most interesting trials was ISIS-3, comparing anistreplase with streptokinase with duteplase.[287] What was

---

[283] For example, ISIS-3.

[284] Hampton (1996).

[285] Continuous Infusion versus Double-Bolus Administration of Alteplase (COBALT) Investigators. (1997). Further details at: http://content.nejm.org/cgi/content/full/338/8/545 (visited 23 May 2005).

[286] AIMS Trial Study Group (1988).

[287] ISIS-3 [Third International Study of Infarct Survival] Collaborative Group (1992).

extraordinary was the superimposition of the three blinds that made it appear as if those three drugs were equal. Now I think that's absolutely amazing because, as was apparent from GUSTO, in fact the regime of tPA that was used in ISIS-3 was not optimal we now know, and the regime used of anistreplase was also not optimal. But the fact that they were superimposed meant that there were suboptimal of the two comparative drugs with streptokinase and they were identical. It seems to me to be quite extraordinary, and I think if the trial had been done with the optimal doses of the two other drugs, the results would have been quite different. I have a recollection that INJECT was actually on reteplase, and not on alteplase.

Quinn: This isn't an original observation. Brian and I discussed this on the phone the other day, but I wonder if we had spent as much money as the pharmaceutical companies do on drug development, on developing ways of getting streptokinase into people an hour sooner, whether we would have seen much more benefit from that drug. That's not an original comment, I know someone, it may be someone like John Rawles, who wrote that, but it's worth throwing into the discussion.[288]

Smith: What's interesting in the days of threats from the Government and minor audit figures in the newspapers, is that if you took part in a trial you added 20 minutes to your door-to-needle time, so we could have done even better in the trial if we didn't have quite difficult randomization. I think it shouldn't go without saying that it was a great privilege to work with the Nottingham group and Bob Wilcox and Professor Hampton really forged a quite remarkable group of collaborators in the UK that started with ASSET, and the development of TRENT, and which developed into a very large number of district general hospitals in the UK that provided large numbers of patients. That was important too, wasn't it, large numbers of patients from each centre into good quality trials. It did something very important, certainly for me as a young consultant trying to get things to be as good as they could be, and that was that the trials imposed an enormous discipline on coronary care units, and also forged something that's talked about a lot today and that is multidisciplinary working, with the nurses and others. I think it had a remarkable effect on cardiology.

Pentecost: We ought to say that streptokinase is only used once, because the antibodies seem to persist almost forever.

---

[288] See, for example, Rawles (1992).

I would still like to discuss the question of the preferred regimen. Should streptokinase be used the first time, because you don't think the differences are very great? Do we still believe there's a slight increase in the risk of stroke with tPA? What's the position with heparin? What has history answered?

References

Abts L R, Beyer R T, Galletti P M, Richardson P D, Karon D, Massimino R, Karlson K E. (1978) Computerized discrimination of microemboli in extracorporeal circuits. *American Journal of Surgery* **135**: 535-8.

Adams J, Heptinstall S, Mitchell J R. (1975) A six-channel automated platelet aggregometer. *Thrombosis et Diathesis Haemorrhagica* **34**: 821–4.

Adams J, Trent R, Rawles J. (1993) Earliest electrocardiographic evidence of myocardial infarction: implications for thrombolytic treatment. The GREAT Group. *British Medical Journal* **307**: 409–13.

AIMS Trial Study Group. (1988) Effect of intravenous APSAC on mortality after acute myocardial infarction: preliminary report of a placebo-controlled clinical trial. AIMS Trial Study Group. *Lancet* **i**: 545–9.

AIMS. (1990) Long-term effects of intravenous anistreplase in acute myocardial infarction: final report of the AIMS study. AIMS Trial Study Group. *Lancet* **335**: 427–31.

Alabaster V A. (1971) Metabolism of vaso-active substances by the lung. PhD thesis, University of London, May 1971.

Alabaster V A, Bakhle Y S. (1970) Removal of 5-hydroxytryptamine in the pulmonary circulation of rat isolated lungs. *British Journal of Pharmacology* **40**: 468–82.

Anonymous. (1958) In Memoriam: Lord Webb-Johnson. *Annals of the Royal College of Surgeons of England* **23**: 64–6.

Anonymous. (1964) Obituary: M J Cross. *British Medical Journal* **ii**: 316.

Anonymous [attributed to Richard Peto]. (1980) Editorial: Aspirin after myocardial infarction. *Lancet* **i**: 1172–3.

Anonymous. (2004) Obituary: Sir John Vane. *Daily Telegraph* (22 November 2004).

Anonymous. (2005) Obituary: Sir John Dacie. *Daily Telegraph* (19 February 2005).

Antiplatelet Trialists' Collaboration. (1994) Collaborative overview of randomized trials of antiplatelet therapy. 1. Prevention of death, myocardial infarction, and stroke by prolonged antiplatelet therapy in various categories of patients. *British Medical Journal* **308**: 81–106. Erratum, *British Medical Journal* **308**: 1540.

Ashby B, Daniel J L, Kitzen J M. (2005) Obituary: J Bryan Smith PhD 1942–2005. *The Pharmacologist* **47**: 78–9. Also available at: www.aspet.org/public/The_Pharmacologist/v47n2_6_05.pdf (visited 21 June 2005).

Avery O T, MacLeod C M, McCarty M. (1944) Studies on the chemical nature of the substance inducing transformation of pneumococcal types. *Journal of Experimental Medicine* **79**: 137–58.

Baigent C, Collins R, Appleby P, Parish S, Sleight P, Peto R. (1998) ISIS-2: Ten year survival among patients with suspected acute myocardial infarction in randomized comparison of intravenous streptokinase, oral aspirin, both, or neither. The ISIS-2 (Second International Study of Infarct Survival) Collaborative Group. *British Medical Journal* **316**: 1337–43.

Barthelemy R, Galletti P M, Trudell L A, MacAndrew J, Richardson P D, Puel P, Enjalbert A. (1982) Total extracorporeal CO2 removal in a pumpless artery-to-vein shunt. *Transactions – American Society for Artificial Internal Organs* **28**: 354–8.

Begent N, Born G V R. (1970) Growth rate *in vivo* of platelet thrombi, produced by iontophoresis of ADP, as a function of mean blood flow velocity. *Nature* **227**: 926–30.

Begent N, Born G V R. (1983) Further evidence that haemostasis depends more on ADP than on thromboxane A_2 in the rat. *Journal of Physiology* **341**: 36P.

Begent N A, Zawilska K, Born G V R. (1983) Novel bleeding time models for quantifying platelet reactions and inhibiting drugs *in vivo*. Standardization of animal models of thrombosis. In Breddin K, Zimmerman R. (eds) *Angiological Symposium Kitzbuhel Proceedings*. Stuttgart; New York, NY: F K Schattauer Verlag, 75–80.

Begent N A, Shafi S, Thorngren M, Born G V R. (1984) Increased bleeding time associated with decreased vascular contractility in rats fed polyunsaturated lipids. *Journal of Physiology* **349**: 69P.

Beswick A D, O'Brien J R, Limb E S, Yarnell J W G, Elwood P C. (1994) Shear-induced filter blockage. A population-based appraisal of a method for the assessment of platelet, white cell and von Willebrand factor interactions. *Platelets* **5**: 186–92.

Biggs R, Douglas A S, Macfarlane R G, Dacie J V, Pitney W R, Merskey C, O'Brien J R. (1952) Christmas disease: a condition previously mistaken for haemophilia. *British Medical Journal* **ii**: 1378–82.

Blaschko H K F. (1983) A biochemist's approach to autopharmacology, in Semenza G (ed.), *Selected Topics in the History of Biochemistry: Personal Recollections.* Comprehensive biochemistry series, vol. 35. Amsterdam: Elsevier, 189–231.

Blaschko H K F, (1985) Ulf Svante von Euler. *Biographical Memoirs of Fellows of the Royal Society* **31**: 143–70.

Blaschko H, Born G V R, D'Iorio A, Eade N R. (1956) Observations on the distribution of catecholamines and adenosine triphosphate in the bovine adrenal medulla. *Journal of Physiology* **133**: 548–57.

Bloom A L, Thomas D P. (eds) (1987) *Haemostasis and Thrombosis.* 2nd edn. Edinburgh; New York, NY: Churchill Livingstone.

Born G V R. (1956a) Adenosine triphosphate (ATP) in blood platelets. *Biochemical Journal* **62**: 33P.

Born G V R. (1956b) The breakdown of adenosine triphosphate in blood platelets during clotting. *Journal of Physiology* **133**: 61–2.

Born G V R. (1962a) Quantitative investigations into the aggregation of blood platelets. *Journal of Physiology* **162**: P67–P68.

Born G V R. (1962b) Aggregation of blood platelets by adenosine diphosphate and its reversal. *Nature* **194**: 927–9.

Born G V R. (1964a) Strong inhibition by 2-chloroadenosine of the aggregation of blood platelets by adenosine diphosphate. *Nature* **202**: 95–6.

Born G V R. (1964b) Obituary: Dr M J Cross. *Nature* **203**: 1013–14.

Born G V R. (1965) Platelets in thrombogenesis: mechanism and inhibition of platelet aggregation. *Annals of the Royal College of Surgeons of England* **36**: 200–6.

Born G V R. (1970) Observations on the change in shape of blood platelets brought about by adenosine diphosphate. *Journal of Physiology* **209**: 487–511.

Born G V R. (1977) *Citation Classic*: Aggregation of blood platelets by adenosine-diphosphate and its reversal. *Current Contents/Life Sciences* (**37**): 8. Also freely available at http://garfield.library.upenn.edu/classics1977/A1977DS89200002.pdf (visited 30 September 2004).

Born G V R. (1985) Adenosine diphosphate as a mediator of platelet aggregation *in vivo*. *Advances in Experimental Medicine and Biology* **192**: 399–409.

Born G V R. (1989) Platelet aggregometry is 25 years old: A *Citation Classic* commentary on the aggregation of blood platelets by Born G V R, Cross M J. *Current Contents/Life Sciences* (**19**): 20. Also freely available at: http://garfield.library.upenn.edu/classics1989/A1989U310000001.pdf (visited 30 September 2004).

Born G V R. (2002a) Afterword: Platelets, a personal story, in Gresele *et al.* (eds) (2002) 1063–72.

Born G V R. (2002b) *The Born Family in Göttingen and Beyond.* Göttingen: Institut fur Wissenschaftsgeschichte.

Born G V R. (2003a) Update on platelets: a personal story (April 2003). *Platelets* **14**: 333-4.

Born G V R. (2003b). Letter to the Editor. *Platelets* **14**: 333–4.

Born G V R, Cross M J. (1963a) Inhibition of the aggregation of blood platelets by substances related to adenosine diphosphate. *Journal of Physiology* **166**: 29P–30P.

Born G V R, Cross M J. (1963b) The aggregation of blood platelets. *Journal of Physiology* **168**: 179–95.

Born G V R, Cross M J. (1964) Effects of inorganic ions and of plasma proteins on the aggregation of blood platelets by adenosine diphosphate. *Journal of Physiology* **170**: 397–414.

Born G V R, Philp R B. (1965) Effects of adenosine analogues and of heparin on platelet thrombi in non-lipaemic and lipaemic rats. *British Journal of Experimental Pathology* **46**: 569–76.

Born G V R, Hume M. (1967) Effects of the numbers and sizes of platelet aggregates on the optical density of plasma. *Nature* **215**: 1027–9.

Born G V R, Kratzer M A. (1984) Source and concentration of extracellular adenosine triphosphate during haemostasis in rats, rabbits and man. *Journal of Physiology* **354**: 419–29.

Born G V R, Richardson P D. (1980) Activation time of blood platelets. *Journal of Membrane Biology* **57**: 87–90.

Born G V R, Honour A J, Mitchell J R A. (1964). Inhibition by adenosine and by 2-chloroadenosine of the formation and embolization of platelet thrombi. *Nature* **202**: 761–5.

Born G V R, Haslam R J, Goldman M. (1965) Comparative effectiveness of adenosine analogues as inhibitors of blood-platelet aggregation and as vasodilators in man. *Nature* **205**: 678–80.

Born G V R, Dearnley R, Foulks J G, Sharp D E. (1978) Quantification of the morphological reaction of platelets to aggregating agents and of its reversal by aggregation inhibitors. *Journal of Physiology* **280**: 193–212.

Born G V R, Cusack H J, Darwin C, McClure M. (1986) Prolongation of bleeding time in rats by ADP receptor antagonists. *Journal of Physiology* **381**: 22P.

Born G V R, Medina R, Shafi S, Cardona-Sanclemente L E. (2003) Factors influencing the uptake of atherogenic plasma proteins by artery walls. *Biorheology* **40**: 13–22.

Bounameaux Y, Roskam J. (1959) [The coupling of platelets with subendothelial fibers]. French. *Comptes Rendus des Seances de la Societe de Biologie et de ses Filiales* **153**: 865–7.

Bowie E J W, Thompson J H Jr, Pascuzzi C A, Owen C A Jr. (1963) Thrombosis in Systemic Lupus Erythematosus despite circulating anticoagulants. *Journal of Laboratory and Clinical Medicine* **62**: 416–30.

Breddin K. (1967) Experimental and clinical investigations on the adhesion and aggregation of human platelets, in Haanen C, Jürgens J. (eds) (1968): 14–23.

Breddin K, Loew D, Lechner K, Uberla K, Walter E. (1980) Secondary prevention of myocardial infarction: a comparison of acetylsalicylic acid, placebo and phenprocoumon. *Haemostasis* **9**: 325–44.

Bunting S, Moncada S, Needleman P, Vane J R. (1976) Proceedings: Formation of prostaglandin endoperoxides and rabbit aorta contracting substance (RCS) by coupling two enzyme systems. *British Journal of Pharmacology* **56**: 344P–5P.

Burr G O, Burr M M. (1930) On the nature and role of fatty acids essential in nutrition. *Journal of Biological Chemistry* **86**: 587–621.

Caerphilly and Speedwell Collaborative Group. (1984) Caerphilly and Speedwell collaborative heart disease studies. *Journal of Epidemiology and Community Health* **38**: 259–62.

Capone M L, Tacconelli S, Sciulli M G, Grana M, Ricciotti E, Minuz P, Di Gregorio P, Merciaro G, Patrono C, Patrignani P. (2004) Clinical pharmacology of platelet, monocyte, and vascular cyclo-oxygenase inhibition by naproxen and low-dose aspirin in healthy subjects. *Circulation* **109**: 1468–71.

CAPRIE Steering Committee. (1996) A randomized, blinded, trial of clopidogrel versus aspirin in patients at risk of ischaemic events (CAPRIE). *Lancet* **348**: 1329–39.

Cardinal D C, Flower R J. (1979) The 'electronic platelet aggregometer'. *British Journal of Pharmacology* **66**: 138P, published in full as Cardinal and Flower (1980).

Cardinal D C, Flower R J. (1980) The electronic aggregometer: a novel device for assessing platelet behaviour in blood. *Journal of Pharmacological Methods* **3**: 135–58.

Chambers D A. (1995) Forty years of DNA, in Chambers D A (ed.) DNA: The double helix, perspective and prospective at 40 years. *Annals of the New York Academy of Sciences* **758**: 1–11.

Chandrasekharan N V, Dai H, Roos K L, Evanson N K, Tomsik J, Elton T, Simmons D L. (2002) COX-3, a cyclo-oxygenase-1 variant inhibited by acetaminophen and other analgesic/antipyretic drugs: cloning, structure, and expression. *Proceedings of the National Academy of Sciences of the USA* **99**: 13926–31.

Chantler C. (2002) The second greatest benefit to mankind? *Lancet* **360**: 1870–7.

Charman W N, Charman S A, Monkhouse D C, Frisbee S E, Lockhart E A, Weisman S, FitzGerald G A. (1993) Biopharmaceutical characterisation of a low-dose (75mg) controlled-release aspirin formulation. *British Journal of Clinical Pharmacology* **36**: 470–3.

Chazov E I. (1965) [Plasmin and streptokinase in the treatment of myocardial infarction]. German. *Zeitschrift für die gesamte innere Medizin und ihre Grenzgebiete* **20**: 727–30.

Chazov E I, Mazaev A V, Torchilin V P, Lebedev B S, Il'ina E V. (1977) [Experimental study of bioresolving preparations of immobilized fibrinolysin]. Russian. *Kardiologiia* **17**: 139–42.

Chelliah R, Bakhle Y S. (1983) The fate of adenine nucleotides in the pulmonary circulation of isolated lung. *Quarterly Journal of Experimental Physiology* **68**: 289–300.

Christie D A, Tansey E M. (eds) (2003) Leukaemia. *Wellcome Witnesses to Twentieth Century Medicine,* vol. 15. London: Wellcome Trust Centre for the History of Medicine at UCL. Freely available online under publications at www.ucl.ac.uk/histmed

Clayton S, Born G V R, Cross M J. (1963) Inhibition of the aggregation of blood platelets by nucleosides. *Nature* **200**: 138–9.

Cleland W P, Bentall H H, Melrose D G, Goodwin J F, Oakley C M, Hollman A. (1968) A decade of open heart surgery. *Lancet* **i**: 191–8.

Cochrane A L. (1976) The development of epidemiology in MRC Units in Wales (1945–75): A personal view. *Journal of the Royal College of Physicians* **10**: 316–20.

Collier H O J. (1969) A pharmacological analysis of aspirin. *Advances in Pharmacology and Chemotherapy* 7: 333–405.

Collier J G, Flower R J. (1971) Effect of aspirin on human seminal prostaglandins. *Lancet* **ii**: 852–3.

Collins R, Scrimgeour A, Yusuf S, Peto R. (1988) Reduction in fatal pulmonary embolism and venous thrombosis by perioperative administration of subcutaneous heparin. Overview of results of randomized trials in general, orthopedic, and urologic surgery. *New England Journal of Medicine* **318**: 1162–73.

Conrad S A, Zwischenberger J B, Grier L R, Alpard S K, Bidani A. (2001) Total extracorporeal arteriovenous carbon dioxide removal in acute respiratory failure: a phase I clinical study. *Intensive Care Medicine* **27**: 1340–51.

Continuous Infusion versus Double-Bolus Administration of Alteplase (COBALT) Investigators. (1997) A comparison of continuous infusion of alteplase with double-bolus administration for acute myocardial infarction. *New England Journal of Medicine* **337**: 1124–30.

Couser W G. (2003) In Memorium: Belding H Scribner, MD. *Kidney International* **64**: 1155–6.

Coyle A J, Page C P, Atkinson L, Flanagan R, Metzger W J. (1990) The requirement for platelets in allergen-induced late asthmatic airways obstruction. Eosinophil infiltration and heightened airway responsiveness in allergic rabbits. *American Review of Respiratory Disease* **142**: 587–93.

Craven L L. (1950) Acetylsalicylic acid, possible preventive of coronary thrombosis. *Annals of Western Medicine and Surgery* **4**: 95–9.

Craven L L. (1953) Experiences with aspirin (acetylsalicylic acid) in the nonspecific prophylaxis of coronary thrombosis. *Mississippi Valley Medical Journal* 75: 38–44. Reproduced as Appendix 2.

Craven L L. (1956) Prevention of coronary thrombosis and cerebral thrombosis. *Mississippi Valley Medical Journal* **78**: 213–5.

Cross M J. (1964) Effect of fibrinogen on the aggregation of platelets by adenosine diphosphate. *Thrombosis et Diathesis Haemorrhagica* **12**: 524–7.

Dacie J. (1979) Evolution of ideas on the life-span of the red blood cell. *Journal of the Royal Society of Medicine* 72: 447–52.

Debre R, Bernard J, Soulier J P, Buhot S, Beaumont J L, Lagrue G. (1952) [A new case of congenital thrombocytic hemorrhagic dystrophy]. *La Presse Medicale* **60**: 1271–4.

De Caterina R, Giannessi D, Bernini W, Gazzetti P, Michelassi C, L'Abbate A, Donato L, Patrignani P, Filabozzi P, Patrono C. (1985) Low-dose aspirin in patients recovering from myocardial infarction. Evidence for a selective inhibition of thromboxane-related platelet function. *European Heart Journal* **6**: 409–17.

de Maat M P, Trion A. (2004) C-reactive protein as a risk factor versus risk marker. *Current Opinion in Lipidology* **15**: 651–7.

Dempster W J, Melrose D G, Bentall H H. (1968) Scientific, technical, and ethical considerations in cardiac transplantation. *British Medical Journal* **i**: 177–8.

Dewar H A. (1979) Acute lysis of coronary thrombi, in Davidson J F. (ed.) *Progress in Chemical Fibrinolysis and Thrombolysis*, vol. 4. Edinburgh: Churchill Livingstone, 273–9.

Dewar H A. (1998) *The Story of Cardiology in Newcastle*. Bishop Auckland: Durham Academic Press.

Dewar H A, Horler A R, Cassells-Smith A J. (1961) Fibrinolytic treatment of coronary thrombosis. A pilot study. *British Medical Journal* **ii**: 671–5.

Dewar H A, Smith R H, Hacking P M. (1978) Rapid lysis of coronary thrombi. The Proceedings of the British Cardiac Society and the Swedish Society of Cardiology, Imperial College, 24–25 November 1977. *British Heart Journal* **40**: 436.

Dewar H A, Stephenson P, Horler A R, Cassells-Smith A J, Ellis P A. (1963) Fibrinolytic therapy of coronary thrombosis. Controlled trial of 75 cases. *British Medical Journal* **ii**: 915–20.

Dioguardi N, Lotto A, Levi G F, Rota M, Proto C, Mannucci PM, Rossi P, Lomanto B, Mattei G, Fiorelli G, Agostini A. (1971) Controlled trial of streptokinase and heparin in acute myocardial infarction. *Lancet* **ii**: 891–5.

Duling B R, Berne R M, Born G V R. (1968) Micro-iontophoretic application of vasoactive agents to the microcirculation of the hamster cheek pouch. *Microvascular Research* **1**: 158–73.

Dutton R C, Baier R E, Dedrick R L, Bowman R L. (1968) Initial thrombus formation on foreign surfaces. *Transactions – American Society for Artificial Internal Organs* **14**: 57–62.

Elwood P C, Renaud S, Beswick A D, O'Brien J R, Sweetnam P M. (1998) Platelet aggregation and incident ischaemic heart disease in the Caerphilly cohort. *Heart* **80**: 578–82.

Elwood P C, Renaud S, Sharp D S, Beswick A D, O'Brien J R, Yarnell J W G. (1991) Ischaemic heart disease and platelet aggregation. The Caerphilly Collaborative Heart Disease Study. *Circulation* **83**: 38–44.

Elwood P C, Beswick A D, O'Brien J R, Yarnell J W, Layzell J C, Limb E S. (1993) Inter-relationships between haemostatic tests and the effects of some dietary determinants in the Caerphilly cohort of older men. *Blood Coagulation and Fibrinolysis* **4**: 529–36.

Elwood P C, Pickering J, Yarnell J, O'Brien J R, Ben-Shlomo Y, Bath P. (2003) Bleeding time, stroke and myocardial infarction: the Caerphilly prospective study. *Platelets* **14**: 139–41.

Elwood P C, Beswick A, Pickering J, McCarron P, O'Brien J R, Renaud S R, Flower R J. (2001) Platelet tests in the prediction of myocardial infarction and ischaemic stroke: evidence from the Caerphilly Prospective Study. *British Journal of Haematology* **113**: 514–20.

Elwood P C, Cochrane A L, Burr M L, Sweetnam P M, Williams G, Welsby E, Hughes S J, Renton R. (1974) A randomized-controlled trial of acetylsalicylic acid in the secondary prevention of mortality from myocardial infarction. *British Medical Journal* **i**: 436–40.

EMIP (European Myocardial Infarction Project) Group. (1993) Prehospital thrombolytic therapy in patients with suspected acute myocardial infarction. The European Myocardial Infarction Project Group. *New England Journal of Medicine* **329**: 383–9.

Emmons P R, Harrison M J, Honour A J, Mitchell J R. (1965) Effect of dipyridamole on human platelet behaviour. *Lancet* **ii**: 603–6.

von Euler U S. (1935) Über die spezifische blutdrucksenkende Substanz des menschlichen Prostata- und Samenblasemselretes. *Klinische Wochenschrift* **14**: 1182–3.

von Euler U S. (1936) On the specific vaso-dilating and plain muscle stimulating substances from accessory genital glands in man and certain animals (prostaglandin and vesiglandin). *Journal of Physiology* **88**: 213–34.

von Euler U S. (1982) Prostaglandin, historical remarks. In Holman R. (ed.) *Golden Jubilee International Congress on Essential Fatty Acids and Prostaglandins.* Oxford, New York, NY: Pergamon Press.

European Cooperative Study Group for Streptokinase Treatment in Acute Myocardial Infarction. (1979) Streptokinase in acute myocardial infarction. *New England Journal of Medicine* **301**: 797–802.

Evans G, Packham M A, Nishizawa E E, Mustard J F, Murphy E A. (1968) The effect of acetylsalicyclic acid on platelet function. *Journal of Experimental Medicine* **128**: 877–94.

Ferreira S H, Moncada S. (1971) Inhibition of prostaglandin synthesis augments the effects of sympathetic nerve stimulation on the cat spleen. *British Journal of Pharmacology* **43**: 419P–20P.

Ferreira S H, Moncada S, Vane J R. (1971) Indomethacin and aspirin abolish prostaglandin release from the spleen. *Nature: New Biology* **231**: 237–9.

Fibrinolytic Therapy Trialists' (FTT) Collaborative Group. (1994) Indications for fibrinolytic therapy in suspected acute myocardial infarction: collaborative overview of early mortality and major morbidity results from all randomized trials of more than 1000 patients. Fibrinolytic Therapy Trialists' (FTT) Collaborative Group. *Lancet* **343**: 311–22. Erratum in *Lancet* **343**: 742.

Fletcher A P, Alkjaersig N, Sherry S. (1959a) The maintenance of a sustained thrombolytic state in man. I. Induction and effects. *Journal of Clinical Investigation* **38**: 1096–110.

Fletcher A P, Sherry S, Alkjaersig N, Smyrniotis F E, Jick S. (1959b) The maintenance of a sustained thrombolytic state in man. II. Clinical observations on patients with myocardial infarction and other thromboembolic disorders. *Journal of Clinical Investigation* **38**: 1111–19.

Fox S C, Sasae R, Janson S, May J A, Heptinstall S. (2004) Quantitation of platelet aggregation and microaggregate formation in whole blood by flow cytometry. *Platelets* **15**: 85–93.

Franzosi M G, Mauri F, Pampallona S, Bossi M, Matta F, Farina M L, Tognoni G. (1987) The GISSI Study: further analysis. Italian Group for the Study of Streptokinase in Myocardial. *Circulation* **76**: II.52–6.

Freemantle N, Cleland J, Young P, Mason J, Harrison J. (1999) Beta blockade after myocardial infarction: systematic review and meta regression analysis. *British Medical Journal* **318**: 1730–7.

French J E. (1958) Chapter 9: Thrombosis, in Florey H. (ed.) *General Pathology*, 2nd edn. London: Lloyd-Luke (Medical Books) Ltd, 180–205.

Fulton W F, Sumner D G. (1976) ^{125}I-Labelled fibrinogen, autoradiography, and stereoarteriography in identification of coronary thrombotic occlusion in fatal myocardial infarction. *British Heart Journal* **38**: 880 (abstract).

Gaarder A, Jonsen J, Laland S, Hellem A, Owren P A. (1961) Adenosine diphosphate in red cells as a factor in the adhesiveness of human blood platelets. *Nature* **192**: 531–2.

GISSI (Gruppo Italiano per lo Studio della Streptochinasi nell'Infarto Miocardico). (1986) Effectiveness of intravenous thrombolytic treatment in acute myocardial infarction. Gruppo Italiano per lo Studio della Streptochinasi nell'Infarto Miocardico (GISSI). *Lancet* **i**: 397–402.

GISSI. (1987) Long-term effects of intravenous thrombolysis in acute myocardial infarction: final report of the GISSI study. *Lancet* **ii**: 871–4.

Gordon E L, Pearson J D, Slakey L L. (1986) The hydrolysis of extracellular adenine nucleotides by cultured endothelial cells from pig aorta. Feed-forward inhibition of adenosine production at the cell surface. *Journal of Biological Chemistry* **261**: 15496–507.

Gordon J L, Milner A J. (1976) Blood platelets as multi-functional cells, in Gordon J L. (ed.) *Platelets in Biology and Pathology*. Research monographs in cell and tissue physiology series, vol. 1. Amsterdam: North-Holland Publishing Co., 1–22.

GREAT (Grampian Region Early Anistreplase Trial) Group. (1992) Feasibility, safety, and efficacy of domiciliary thrombolysis by general practitioners: Grampian region early anistreplase trial. *British Medical Journal* **305**: 548–53.

Gresele P, Page C P, Fuster V, Vermylen J. (eds) (2002) *Platelets in Thrombotic and Non-thrombotic Disorders: Pathophysiology, Pharmacology and Therapeutics*. Cambridge and New York, NY: Cambridge University Press.

Grüntzig A, Schneider H J. (1977) [The percutaneous dilatation of chronic coronary stenoses – experiments and morphology]. German. *Schweizerische medizinische Wochenschrift* **107**: 1588. Reports on 225 cases of percutaneous transluminal angioplasty of peripheral arteries performed since 1971.

Gryglewski R, Vane J R. (1972) The generation from arachidonic acid of rabbit aorta contracting substance (RCS) by a microsomal enzyme preparation which also generates prostaglandins. *British Journal of Pharmacology* **46**: 449–57.

GUSTO (Global Utilization of Streptokinase and tPA for Occluded Coronary Arteries) investigators. (1993) An international randomized trial comparing four thrombolytic strategies for acute myocardial infarction. *New England Journal of Medicine* **329**: 673–82.

Haanen C, Jürgens J. (eds) (1968) *Platelets in Haemostasis*. Experimental biology and medicine series, vol. 3, contributions to a conference held at Castel Miemo, near Pisa, in the autumn of 1967. Basel; New York, NY: S Karger.

Hamberg M, Samuelsson B. (1974) Prostaglandin endoperoxides. Novel transformations of arachidonic acid in human platelets. *Proceedings of the National Academy of Sciences of the USA* **71**: 3400–4.

Hamberg M, Svensson J, Samuelsson B. (1975) Thromboxanes: a new group of biologically active compounds derived from prostaglandin endoperoxides. *Proceedings of the National Academy of Sciences of the USA* **72**: 2994–8.

H(ampton) J R. (1991) Obituary: J R A Mitchell. *British Medical Journal* **302**: 843.

Hampton J R. (1996) Mega-trials and equivalence trials: experience from the INJECT study. *European Heart Journal* **17**(Suppl E): 28–34.

Hampton J R, Mitchell J R. (1966) Modification of the electrokinetic response of blood platelets to aggregating agents. *Nature* **210**: 1000–2.

Hampton K K, Cerletti C, Loizou L A, Bucchi F, Donati M B, Davies J A, de Gaetano G, Prentice C R M. (1990) Coagulation, fibrinolytic and platelet function in patients on long-term therapy with aspirin 300mg or 1200mg daily compared with placebo. *Thrombosis and Haemostasis* **64**: 17–20.

Hankey G J, Eikelboom J W. (2004) Aspirin resistance. *British Medical Journal* **328**: 477–9.

Hardaway R M III, McKay D G. (1959) Disseminated intravascular coagulation: a cause of shock. *Annals of Surgery* **149**: 462–70.

Hardisty R M. (1977) Disorders of platelet function. *British Medical Bulletin* **33**: 207–12.

Hardisty R M. (1983) Hereditary disorders of platelet function. *Clinics in Haematology* **12**: 153–73.

Hardman J G, Limbird L E. (eds) (2001) *Goodman and Gilman's The Pharmacological Basis of Therapeutics*. 10th edn. New York, NY: McGraw-Hill.

Harrison M J, Marshall J, Meadows J C, Russell R W. (1971) Effect of aspirin in amaurosis fugax. *Lancet* **ii**: 743–4.

Harrison S, Geppetti P. (2001) Substance P. *International Journal of Biochemistry and Cell Biology* **33**: 555–76.

Heath H, Brigden W D, Canever J V, Pollock J, Hunter P R, Kelsey J, Bloom A. (1971) Platelet adhesiveness and aggregation in relation to diabetic retinopathy. *Diabetologia* 7: 308–15.

Hellem A J. (1960) The adhesiveness of human blood platelets *in vitro*. *Scandinavian Journal of Clinical and Labatory Investigation* **12**(Suppl): 1–117.

Hennekens C H, Eberlein K. (1985) A randomized trial of aspirin and β-carotene among US physicians. *Preventive Medicine* 14: 165–8.

Hennekens C H, Peto R, Hutchison G B, Doll R. (1988) Letter: An overview of the British and American aspirin studies. *New England Journal of Medicine* **318**: 923–4.

Hill J D, O'Brien T G, Murray J J, Dontigny L, Bramson M L, Osborn J J, Gerbode F. (1972) Extracorporeal oxygenation for acute post-traumatic respiratory failure (shock-lung syndrome): use of the Bramson membrane lung. *New England Journal of Medicine* **286**: 629–34.

Hillmen P, Lewis S M, Bessler M, Luzzatto L, Dacie J V. (1995) Natural history of paroxysmal nocturnal hemoglobinuria. *New England Journal of Medicine* **333**: 1253–8.

Hirsh J, Dalen J E, Fuster V, Harker L B, Patrono C, Roth G. (1995) Aspirin and other platelet-active drugs. The relationship among dose, effectiveness, and side effects. *Chest* **108**: 247S–57S.

Hlatky M A, Bacon C, Boothroyd D, Mahanna E, Reves J G, Newman M F, Johnstone I, Winston C, Brooks M M, Rosen A D, Mark D B, Pitt B, Rogers W, Ryan T, Wiens R, Blumenthal J A. (1997) Cognitive function five years after randomization to coronary angioplasty or coronary artery bypass graft surgery. *Circulation* **96**(Suppl): II.11–14; discussion II.15.

Hollaender A, Freireich E J. (1965) Symposium: Second Conference on Blood Platelets; In Memorium. *Blood* **25**: 597–613.

Honour A J, Mitchell J R A. (1964) Platelet clumping in injured vessels. *British Journal of Experimental Pathology* **45**: 75–87.

Hook E B. (ed.) (2002) *Prematurity in Scientific Discovery: On resistance and neglect.* Berkeley, CA; London: University of California Press.

Hourani S M, Cusack N J. (1991) Pharmacological receptors on blood platelets. *Pharmacological Reviews* **43**: 243–98.

Hugenholtz P G, Rentrop P. (1982) Thrombolytic therapy for acute myocardial infarction: *quo vadis?* A review of the recent literature. *European Heart Journal* **3**: 395–403.

Hughes G R V. (1993) The antiphospholipid syndrome: ten years on. *Lancet* **342**: 341–4.

ISIS (International Study of Infarct Survival). (1987) Randomized factorial trial of high-dose intravenous streptokinase, of oral aspirin and of intravenous heparin in acute myocardial infarction. ISIS pilot study. *European Heart Journal* **8**: 634–42.

ISIS-2 (Second International Study of Infarct Survival). (1988) Randomized trial of intravenous streptokinase, oral aspirin, both, or neither among 17 187 cases of suspected acute myocardial infarction: ISIS-2. *Lancet* **ii**: 349–60. See also Comment in *Lancet*, 1997, **349**: 1551.

ISIS-3 (Third International Study of Infarct Survival) Collaborative Group. (1992) ISIS-3: a randomized comparison of streptokinase *vs* tissue plasminogen activator *vs* anistreplase and of aspirin plus heparin *vs* aspirin alone among 41 299 cases of suspected acute myocardial infarction. Third International Study of Infarct Survival Collaborative Group. *Lancet* **339**: 753–70.

James D M, Born G V R. (1980) Uptake of purine bases and nucleosides in African trypanosomes. *Parasitology* **81**: 383–93.

Jamieson G A, Scipio A R. (eds) (1982) *Interaction of Platelets and Tumor Cells.* Papers from the proceedings of the Chesapeake Conference held at St Mary's College, St Mary's, Maryland, 26–30 June 1981. Progress in clinical and biological research series, vol. 89. New York, NY: Liss.

Jick H, Miettinen O S, Shapiro S, Lewis G P, Siskind V, Slone D. (1970) Comprehensive drug surveillance. *Journal of the American Medical Association* **213**: 1455–60.

Johnson P C, Ware J A, Cliveden P B, Smith M, Dvorak A M, Salzman E W. (1985) Measurement of ionized calcium in blood platelets with the photoprotein aequorin. *Journal of Biological Chemistry* **260**: 2069–76.

Jy W, Horstman L L, Homolak D, Ahn Y S. (1995) Electrophoretic properties of platelets from normal, thrombotic and ITP patients by doppler electrophoretic light scattering analysis. *Platelets* **6**: 354–8.

Kennedy J W, Fritz J K, Ritchie J L. (1982) Streptokinase in acute myocardial infarction: western Washington randomized trial – protocol and progress report. *American Heart Journal* **104**: 899–911.

Kennedy J W, Ritchie J L, Davis K B, Fritz J K. (1983) Western Washington randomized trial of intracoronary streptokinase in acute myocardial infarction. *New England Journal of Medicine* **309**: 1477–82.

Kennedy J W, Ritchie J L, Davis K B, Stadius M L, Maynard C, Fritz J K. (1985) The western Washington randomized trial of intracoronary streptokinase in acute myocardial infarction. A 12-month follow-up report. *New England Journal of Medicine* **312**: 1073–8.

Kortenhaus H, Schroer H, Born G V R. (1982) Quantification of the adhesion of platelets in hamster venules *in vivo. Proceedings of the Royal Society of London. Series B* **215**: 135–45.

Kratzer M A, Born G V R. (1985) Simulation of primary haemostasis *in vitro. Haemostasis* **15**: 357–62.

Latimer P, Born G V R, Michal F. (1977) Application of light-scattering theory to the optical effects associated with the morphology of blood platelets. *Archives of Biochemistry and Biophysics* **180**: 151–9.

Leininger R I, Cooper C W, Falb R D, Grode G A. (1966) Nonthrombogenic plastic surfaces. *Science* **152**: 1625–6.

Leonard E F, Turitto V T, Vroman L. (eds) (1987) *Blood in Contact with Natural and Artificial Surfaces,* Annals of the New York Academy of Sciences series, vol. 516. New York, NY: New York Academy of Sciences.

Lewis C, Elwood P C. (2002) Obituary: John O'Brien (1915–2002). *Guardian* (11 December 2002).

Liebold A, Reng C M, Philipp A, Pfeifer M, Birnbaum D E. (2000) Pumpless extracorporeal lung assist – experience with the first 20 cases. *European Journal of Cardiothoracic Surgery* **17**: 608–13.

Loewi O. (1953) *From the Workshop of Discoveries.* Lawrence, KS: University of Kansas Press.

Macfarlane G. (1979) *Howard Florey: The making of a great scientist.* Oxford; New York, NY: Oxford University Press.

Macmillan D C. (1966) Secondary clumping effect in human citrated platelet-rich plasma produced by adenosine diphosphate and adrenaline. *Nature* **211**: 140–4.

Macmillan D C, Oliver M F. (1965) The initial changes in platelet morphology following the addition of adenosine diphosphate. *Journal of Atherosclerosis Research* **20**: 440–4.

Maddox B. (2002) *Rosalind Franklin: The dark lady of DNA.* London: HarperCollins.

Mahaut-Smith M P, Sage S O, Rink T J. (1990) Receptor-activated single channels in intact human platelets. *Journal of Biological Chemistry* **265**: 10479–83.

Mahaut-Smith M P, Ennion S J, Rolf M G, Evans R J. (2000) ADP is not an agonist at P2X1 receptors: evidence for separate receptors stimulated by ATP and ADP on human platelets. *British Journal of Pharmacology* **131**: 108–14.

Mahaut-Smith M P, Thomas D, Higham A B, Usher-Smith J A, Hussain J F, Martinez-Pinna J, Skepper J N, Mason M J. (2003) Properties of the demarcation membrane system in living rat megakaryocytes. *Biophysical Journal* **84**: 2646–54.

Majerus P W, Tollefsen D M. (2001) Anticoagulant, thrombolytic and antiplatelet drugs, in Hardman and Limbird (eds) (2001), 1519–38.

Martin J F, Bath P M, Burr M L. (1991) Influence of platelet size on outcome after myocardial infarction. *Lancet* **338**: 1409–11.

Maruyama Y. (1987) A patch-clamp study of mammalian platelets and their voltage-gated potassium current. *Journal of Physiology* **391**: 467–85.

McCarthy L J, Dlott J S, Orazi A, Waxman D, Miraglia C C, Danielson C F. (2004) Thrombotic thrombocytopenic purpura: yesterday, today, tomorrow. *Therapeutic Apheresis and Dialysis* **8**: 80–6.

McGill H C Jr, McMahan C A, Herderick E E, Malcom G T, Tracy R E, Strong J P. (2000) Origin of atherosclerosis in childhood and adolescence. *American Journal of Clinical Nutrition* **72**(5 Suppl): 1307S–15S.

McLean R F, Wong B I, Naylor C D, Snow W G, Harrington E M, Gawel M, Fremes S E. (1994) Cardiopulmonary bypass, temperature, and central nervous system dysfunction. *Circulation* **90**(5 Pt 2): II.250–5.

McNicol G P, Douglas A S. (1964) Epsilon-aminocaproic acid and other inhibitors of fibrinolysis. *British Medical Bulletin* **20**: 233–9.

McNicol G P, Douglas A S. (1967) Platelet abnormality in human scurvy. *Lancet* **i**: 975–8.

Meade T W, North W R, Chakrabarti R R, Stirling Y, Haines A P, Thompson S G, Brozovic M. (1980) Haemostatic function and cardiovascular death: early results of a prospective study. *Lancet* **i**: 1050–4.

Meade T W, Mellows S, Brozovic M, Miller G J, Chakrabarti R R, North W R, Haines A P, Stirling Y, Imeson J D, Thompson S G. (1986) Haemostatic function and ischaemic heart disease: principal results of the Northwick Park Heart Study. *Lancet* **ii**: 533–7.

Meier B, Rutishauser W. (1985) Transluminal coronary angioplasty – state of the art 1984. *Acta Medica Scandinavica Supplementum* **701**: 142-7.

Melrose D G (1953) Mechanical heart–lung for use in man. *British Medical Journal* **ii**: 57–62.

Melrose D G, Bassett J W, Beaconsfield P, Graber I G, Shackman R. (1953) Experimental physiology of a heart–lung machine in parallel with normal circulation. *British Medical Journal* **ii**: 62–6.

Merx W, Dorr R, Rentrop P, Blanke H, Karsch K R, Mathey D G, Kremer P, Rutsch W, Schmutzler H. (1981) Evaluation of the effectiveness of intracoronary streptokinase infusion in acute myocardial infarction: postprocedure management and hospital course in 204 patients. *American Heart Journal* **102**: 1181–7.

Michal F, Born G V R. (1971) Effect of the rapid shape change of platelets on the transmission and scattering of light through plasma. *Nature: New biology* **231**: 220–2.

Millar K, Asbury A J, Murray G D. (2001) Pre-existing cognitive impairment as a factor influencing outcome after cardiac surgery. *British Journal of Anaesthesia* **86**: 63–7.

Mills D C B, Robb I A, Roberts G C K. (1968) The release of nucleotides, 5-hydroxytryptamine and enzymes from human blood platelets during aggregation. *Journal of Physiology* **195**: 715–29.

Mitchell J R A. (1959) Inhibition of heparin clearing by platelets. *Lancet* **i**: 169–72.

Mitchell J R A, for GRAND (Glaxo Receptor Antagonist against Nottingham DVT) Study Group. (1987) *Trial of thromboxane receptor antagonist as prophylaxis against deep vein thrombosis in suspected acute myocardial infarction.* Uxbridge, Middlesex: Glaxo [Glaxo internal report].

Moncada S. (2005) Obituary: Sir John Vane. *Nature* **433**: 28.

Moncada S, Gryglewski R, Bunting S, Vane J R. (1976) An enzyme isolated from arteries transforms prostaglandin endoperoxides to an unstable substance that inhibits platelet aggregation. *Nature* **263**: 663–5.

Moncada S, Bunting S, Mullane K, Thorogood P, Vane J R, Raz A, Needleman P. (1977) Imidazole: a selective inhibitor of thromboxane synthetase. *Prostaglandins* **13**: 611–18.

Morley J. (1977) Prostaglandins and the lung. *Postgraduate Medical Journal* **53**: 652–3.

Morris C D W. (1967) Acetylsalicylic acid and platelet stickiness. *Lancet* **i**: 279–80. Morris wrote from Fa Dr Karl Thomae Gmbh, Biberach, Germany.

Morris C D W, Miller K. (1966) Studies on the modification of a method for determining platelet stickiness. *South African Journal of Medical Sciences* **31**: 45–6.

Morrow J D, Roberts, L J II. (2001a) Lipid-derived autacoids: eicosanoids and platelet-activating factor. Chapter 26 in Hardman and Limbird (2001): 669–85.

Morrow J D, Roberts, L J II. (2001b) Analgesic-antipyretic and anti-inflammatory agents and drugs employed in the treatment of gout. Chapter 27 in Hardman and Limbird (2001): 687–731.

Moschcowitz E. (1925) An acute febrile pleiochromic anaemia with hyaline thrombosis of the terminal arterioles and capillaries. *Archives of Internal Medicine* **36**: 89–93.

Mustard J F, Packham M A. (1970) Factors influencing platelet function: adhesion, release, and aggregation. *Pharmacological Reviews* **22**: 97–187.

Mustard J F, Packham M A. (1977) Normal and abnormal haemostasis. *British Medical Bulletin* **33**: 187–92.

Mustard J F, Glynn M F, Nishizawa E E, Packham M A. (1967) Platelet surface interactions: relationship to thrombosis and hemostasis. *Federation Proceedings* **26**: 106–14.

Needleman P, Moncada S, Bunting S, Vane J R, Hamberg M, Samuelsson B. (1976) Identification of an enzyme in platelet microsomes which generates thromboxane A_2 from prostaglandin endoperoxides. *Nature* **261**: 558–60.

Ness A R, Reynolds L A, Tansey E M. (eds) (2002) Population-based Research in South Wales: The MRC Pneumoconiosis Research Unit and the MRC Epidemiology Unit. *Wellcome Witnesses to Twentieth Century Medicine*, vol. 13. London: The Wellcome Trust Centre for the History of Medicine at UCL. Freely available online under publications at www.ucl.ac.uk/histmed

Nilsson I M. (1994) [Haemophilia–then and now]. Swedish. *Sydsven Medicinhist Sallsk Arsskr* **31**: 33–52.

Nilsson I M, Blomback M, Jorpes E, Blomback B, Johansson S A. (1957) Von Willebrand's disease and its correction with human plasma fraction 1–0. *Acta Medica Scandinavica* **159**: 179–88.

Norris R M, White H D. (1988) Therapeutic trials in coronary thrombosis should measure left ventricular function as primary end-point of treatment. *Lancet* **i**: 104–6.

Norris R M, Agnew T M, Brandt P W, Graham K J, Hill D G, Kerr A R, Lowe J B, Roche A H, Whitlock R M, Barratt-Boyes B G. (1981) Coronary surgery after recurrent myocardial infarction: progress of a trial comparing surgical with nonsurgical management for asymptomatic patients with advanced coronary disease. *Circulation* **63**: 785–92.

Norwegian Multicentre Study Group. (1981) Timolol-induced reduction in mortality and reinfarction in patients surviving acute myocardial infarction. *New England Journal of Medicine* **304**: 801–7.

Nose Y, Kwan-Gett C S, Hino K, Kolff W J, Effler D B. (1967) Clot formation inside the artificial heart device. *Journal of Thoracic and Cardiovascular Surgery* **54**: 697–706.

O'Brien J R. (1962) Platelet aggregation Part II. Some results from a new method of study. *Journal of Clinical Pathology* **15**: 452–5.

O'Brien J R. (1968a) Aspirin and platelet aggregation. *Lancet* **i**: 204–5.

O'Brien J R. (1968b) Effects of salicylates on human platelets. *Lancet* **i**: 779–83.

O'Brien J R, Salmon G P. (1990) An independent haemostatic mechanism: shear induced platelet aggregation. *Advances in Experimental Medicine and Biology* **281**: 287–96.

O'Rourke M, Baron D, Keogh A, Kelly R, Nelson G, Barnes C, Raftos J, Graham K, Hillman K, Newman H. (1988) Limitation of myocardial infarction by early infusion of recombinant tissue-type plasminogen activator. *Circulation* 77: 1311–5.

Page C P, Paul W, Morley J. (1982) An *in vivo* model for studying platelet aggregation and disaggregation. *Thrombosis and Haemostasis* 47: 210–13.

Palmer R M, Ferrige A G, Moncada S. (1987) Nitric oxide release accounts for the biological activity of endothelium-derived relaxing factor. *Nature* **327**: 524–6.

Patrono C, Coller B, Dalen J E, Fuster V, Gent M, Harker L A, Hirsh J, Roth G. (1998) Platelet-active drugs: the relationships among dose, effectiveness, and side effects. *Chest* **114**(5 Suppl): 470S–88S.

Patrono C, Coller B, Dalen J E, FitzGerald G A, Fuster V, Gent M, Hirsh J, Roth G. (2001) Platelet-active drugs: the relationships among dose, effectiveness, and side effects. *Chest* **119**(1 Suppl): 39S–63S.

Payne D A, Jones C I, Hayes P D, Webster S E, Ross Naylor A, Goodall A H. (2004) Platelet inhibition by aspirin is diminished in patients during carotid surgery: a form of transient aspirin resistance? *Thrombosis and Haemostasis* **92**: 89–96.

Peto R, Gray R, Collins R, Wheatley K, Hennekens C, Jamrozik K, Warlow C, Hafner B, Thompson E, Norton S, Gilliland J, Doll R. (1988) Randomized trial of prophylactic daily aspirin in British male doctors. *British Medical Journal* **296**: 313–16.

Physicians' Health Study Research Group, Steering Committee. (1989) Final report on the aspirin component of the ongoing Physicians' Health Study. *New England Journal of Medicine* **321**: 129–35.

Piper P J, Vane J R. (1969) Release of additional factors in anaphylaxis and its antagonism by anti-inflammatory drugs. *Nature* **223**: 29–35.

Pitchford S C, Riffo-Vasquez Y, Sousa A, Momi S, Gresele P, Spina D, Page C P. (2004) Platelets are necessary for airway wall remodelling in a murine model of chronic allergic inflammation. *Blood* **103**: 639–47.

Pitchford S C, Yano H, Lever R, Riffo-Vasquez Y, Ciferri S, Rose M J, Giannini S, Momi S, Spina D, O'Connor B, Gresele P, Page C P. (2003) Platelets are essential for leukocyte recruitment in allergic inflammation. *Journal of Allergy and Clinical Immunology* **112**: 109–18.

Poliwoda H, Diederich K W, Schneider B, Rodenburg R, Heckner F, Kortge P, van de Loo J, Pezold F A, Praetorius F, Schmutzler R, Zekorn D. (1966) [On the thrombolytic therapy of recent myocardial infarction. 2. Results of electrocardiographic studies]. German. *Deutsche Medizinische Wochenschrift* **91**: 978–84.

Pozzan T, Arslan P, Tsien R Y, Rink T J. (1982) Anti-immunoglobulin, cytoplasmic free calcium, and capping in B lymphocytes. *Journal of Cell Biology* **94**: 335–40.

Prentice C R M, McNicol G P, Douglas A S. (1966) Effect of normal and atheromatous aortic tissue on platelet aggregation *in vitro*. *Journal of Clinical Pathology* **19**: 343–7.

Principal Investigators. (1978) A co-operative trial in the primary prevention of ischaemic heart disease using clofibrate. Report from the Committee of Principal Investigators. *British Heart Journal* **40**: 1069–118.

Pulmonary Embolism Prevention (PEP) trial. (2000) Prevention of pulmonary embolism and deep vein thrombosis with low dose aspirin: Pulmonary Embolism Prevention (PEP) trial. *Lancet* **355**: 1295–302

Quick A J. (1966) Salicylates and bleeding: the aspirin tolerance test. *American Journal of the Medical Sciences* **252**: 265–9.

Rapaport E. (1991) Overview: rationale of thrombolysis in treating acute myocardial infarction. *Heart and Lung* **20**: 538–41.

Rapport M M, Green A A, Page I H. (1948) Serum vasoconstrictor (serotonin). IV. Isolation and characterization. *Journal of Biological Chemistry* **176**: 1243–51.

Rawles J M. (1992) Risk–benefit analysis of thrombolytic therapy for acute MI: a perspective. *Coronary Artery Disease* **3**: 1153–61.

Raz A, Wyche A, Siegel N, Needleman P. (1988) Regulation of fibroblast Cyclo-oxygenase synthesis by interleukin-1. *Journal of Biological Chemistry* **263**: 3022–8.

Renaud S, Dumont E, Godsey F, Suplisson A, Thevenon C. (1979) Platelet functions in relation to dietary fats in farmers from two regions of France. *Thrombosis and Haemostasis* **40**: 518–31.

Rentrop P, Blanke H, Kostering H, Karsch K R. (1980) [Intracoronary application of streptokinase in acute myocardial infarction and non-stable angina pectoris (author's transl)]. German. *Deutsche Medizinische Wochenschrift* **105**: 221–8.

Reynolds L A, Tansey E M. (eds). (2000) Clinical Research in Britain, 1958–80. *Wellcome Witnesses to Twentieth Century Medicine,* vol. 7. London: The Wellcome Trust. Freely available online under publications at www.ucl.ac.uk/histmed

Reynolds L A, Tansey E M. (eds). (2004) Innovation in Pain Management. *Wellcome Witnesses to Twentieth Century Medicine,* vol. 21. London: Wellcome Trust Centre for the History of Medicine at UCL. Freely available online under publications at www.ucl.ac.uk/histmed

Richardson P D, Galletti P M, Born G V R. (1976) Regional administration of drugs to control thrombosis in artificial organs. *Transactions – American Society for Artificial Internal Organs* **22**: 22–9.

Ridker P M, Cushman M, Stampfer M J, Tracy R P, Hennekens C H. (1997) Inflammation, aspirin, and the risk of cardiovascular disease in apparently healthy men. *New England Journal of Medicine* **336**: 973–9.

Rink T J. (1982) *Measurement of Membrane Potential with Chemical Probes.* Techniques in lipid and membrane biochemistry series. Shannon: Elsevier Biomed.

Rink T J. (1987) *Stimulus-response Coupling.* MD thesis, University of Cambridge, 20 January 1987.

Rink T J, Smith S W, Tsien R Y. (1982) Cytoplasmic free Ca2+ in human platelets: Ca2+ thresholds and Ca-independent activation for shape-change and secretion. *FEBS Letters* **148**: 21–6.

Robb-Smith A H T. (1967) Why the platelets were discovered. *British Journal of Haematology* **13**: 618–37.

Salzman E W. (1972) Cyclic AMP and platelet function. *New England Journal of Medicine* **286**: 358–63.

Salzman E W. (1976) Prostaglandins and platelet function. *Advances in Prostaglandin and Thromboxane Research* **2**: 767–80.

Salzman E W, Chambers D A. (1964) Inhibition of ADP-induced platelet aggregation by substituted amino-acids. *Nature* **204**: 698–700.

Salzman E W, Chambers D A. (1965) Incorporation by blood platelets of adenosine diphosphate labelled with carbon-14. *Nature* **206**: 727–8.

Salzman E W, Chambers D A, Neri L L. (1966) Possible mechanism of aggregation of blood platelets by adenosine diphosphate. *Nature* **210**: 167–9.

Salzman E W, Ashford T P, Chambers D A, Neri L L, Dempster A P. (1969) Platelet volume: effect of temperature and agents affecting platelet aggregation. *American Journal of Physiology* **217**: 1330–8.

Sharp D S, Beswick A D, O'Brien J R, Renaud S, Yarnell J W, Elwood P C. (1990) The association of platelet and red cell count with platelet impedance changes in whole blood and light-scattering changes in platelet-rich plasma: evidence from the Caerphilly Collaborative Heart Disease Study. *Thrombosis and Haemostasis* **64**: 211–15.

Silman A J. (1986) Recent trends in rheumatoid arthritis. *British Journal of Rheumatology* **25**: 328–30.

Simoons M L, Vos J, Tijssen J G, Vermeer F, Verheugt F W, Krauss X H, Cats V M. (1989) Long-term benefit of early thrombolytic therapy in patients with acute myocardial infarction: five year follow-up of a trial conducted by the Interuniversity Cardiology Institute of The Netherlands. *Journal of the American College of Cardiology* **14**: 1609–15.

Sixty Plus Reinfarction Study Research Group. (1980) A double-blind trial to assess long-term oral anticoagulant therapy in elderly patients after myocardial infarction: report. *Lancet* **ii**: 989–94.

Smith J B. (2004) Aspirin. *Journal of Thrombosis and Haemostasis* **2**: 335–41.

Smith J B, Willis A L. (1971) Aspirin selectively inhibits prostaglandin production in human platelets. *Nature: New Biology* **231**: 235–7.

Smith P, Arnesen H, Holme I. (1990) The effect of warfarin on mortality and reinfarction after myocardial infarction. *New England Journal of Medicine* **323**: 147–52.

Smith W L, DeWitt D L, Garavito R M. (2000) Cyclo-oxygenases: structural, cellular, and molecular biology. *Annual Review of Biochemistry* **69**: 145–82.

Snow P J D. (1965) Effect of propranolol in myocardial infarction. *Lancet* **ii**: 551–3.

Stafford N P, Pink A E, White A E, Glenn J R, Heptinstall S. (2003) Mechanisms involved in adenosine triphosphate-induced platelet aggregation in whole blood. *Arteriosclerosis, Thrombosis, and Vascular Biology* **23**: 1928–33.

Stampfer M J, Goldhaber S Z, Yusuf S, Peto R, Hennekens C H. (1982) Effect of intravenous streptokinase on acute MI: pooled results from randomized trials. *New England Journal of Medicine* **307**: 1180–2.

Starling E H, Verney E B. (1925) The excretion of urine as studied in the isolated kidney. *Proceedings of the Royal Society of London. Series B. Biological sciences* **97**: 321–63.

Stent G S. (1972) Prematurity and uniqueness in scientific discovery. *Scientific American* **227**: 84–93.

Strehler B D, Totter J R. (1954) Determination of ATP and related compounds: firefly luminescence and other methods, in Glick D. (ed.) *Methods of Biochemical Analysis,* vol. 1. London: Interscience, 342–56.

Szczeklik A, Milner P C, Birch J, Watkins J, Martin J F. (1986) Prolonged bleeding time, reduced platelet aggregation, altered PAF-acether sensitivity and increased platelet mass are a trait of asthma and hay fever. *Thrombosis and Haemostasis* **56**: 283–7.

Tansey E M, Christie D A. (eds) (1997) Endogenous opiates, in Tansey E M, Catterall P P, Christie D A, Willhoft S V, Reynolds L A. (eds) *Wellcome Witnesses to Twentieth Century Medicine,* vol. 1. London: The Wellcome Trust, 67–101. Freely available online under publications at www.ucl.ac.uk/histmed

Tansey E M, Christie D A. (eds) (1999) Haemophilia: Recent history of clinical management. *Wellcome Witnesses to Twentieth Century Medicine*, vol. 4. London: The Wellcome Trust. Freely available online under publications at www.ucl.ac.uk/histmed

Tansey E M, Reynolds L A. (eds) (1999) Early heart transplant surgery in the UK. *Wellcome Witnesses to Twentieth Century Medicine*, vol. 3. London: The Wellcome Trust. Freely available online under publications at www.ucl.ac.uk/histmed

Taylor K M. (ed.) (1986) *Cardiopulmonary Bypass: Principles and management.* London: Chapman and Hall.

Thaulow E, Erikssen J, Sandvik L, Stormorken H, Cohn P F. (1991) Blood platelet count and function are related to total and cardiovascular death in apparently healthy men. *Circulation* **84**: 613–17.

Thomas D P. (1972) Abnormalities of platelet aggregation in patients with alcoholic cirrhosis. *Annals of the New York Academy of Sciences* **201**: 243–50.

Thomas D P, Ream V J, Stuart R K. (1967) Platelet aggregation in patients with Laennec's cirrhosis of the liver. *New England Journal of Medicine* **276**: 1344–8.

Thorngren M, Shafi S, Born G V R. (1983a) Thromboxane A_2 in skin-bleeding-time blood and in clotted venous blood before and after administration of acetylsalicylic acid. *Lancet* **i**: 1075–8.

Thorngren M, Shafi S, Born G V R. (1983b) Quantification of blood from skin-bleeding-time determinations: effects of fish diet or acetylsalicylic acid. *Haemostasis* **13**: 282–7.

Thorngren M, Shafi S, Born G V R. (1984) Delay in primary haemostasis produced by a fish diet without change in local thromboxane A_2. *British Journal of Haematology* **58**: 567–78.

Topol E J. (2000) Acute myocardial infarction: thrombolysis. *Heart* **83**: 122–6.

Trip M D, Cats V M, van Capelle F J, Vreeken J. (1990) Platelet hyperreactivity and prognosis in survivors of myocardial infarction. *New England Journal of Medicine* **322**: 1549–54.

Tsien R Y. (1980) New calcium indicators and buffers with high selectivity against magnesium and protons: design, synthesis, and properties of prototype structures. *Biochemistry* **19**: 2396–404.

Tsien R Y, Pozzan T, Rink T J. (1982) Calcium homeostasis in intact lymphocytes: cytoplasmic free calcium monitored with a new, intracellularly trapped fluorescent indicator. *Journal of Cell Biology* **94**: 325–34.

UK-TIA Study Group. (1988) United Kingdom transient ischaemic attack (UK-TIA) aspirin trial: interim results. *British Medical Journal* **296**: 316–20.

Vane J R. (1971) Inhibition of prostaglandin synthesis as a mechanism of action for aspirin-like drugs. *Nature: New Biology* **231**: 232–5.

Vane J R. (1972) Prostaglandins and the aspirin-like drugs. *Hospital Practice*: 61–71.

Vane J R. (1983) Nobel lecture. Adventures and excursions in bioassay – the stepping stones to prostacyclin. *Postgraduate Medical Journal* **59**: 743–58. Also published as Nobel Lecture, 8 December 1982, in Lindsten J. (ed.) (1993) *Nobel Lectures in Physiology or Medicine: 1981–90*. Singapore: World Scientific, 145–70.

Vane J R. (1992) The discovery of drugs and animal research, in Botting J H (ed.) *Animal Experimentation and the Future of Medical Research*. Proceedings of a conference organized by the Research Defence Society on 26 April 1991 at the Royal Society, London. London and Chapel Hill, NC: Portland Press, 39–46.

Vane J R, Bakhle Y S, Botting R M. (1998) Cyclo-oxygenases 1 and 2. *Annual Review of Pharmacology and Toxicology* **38**: 97–120.

Vlodavsky I, Friedmann Y. (2001) Molecular properties and involvement of heparanase in cancer metastasis and angiogenesis. *Journal of Clinical Investigation* **108**: 341–7.

Weatherall D, Lock S. (1997) Roger Michael Hardisty. *British Medical Journal* **315**: 955.

Weiss H J, Aledort L M. (1967) Impaired platelet–connective-tissue reaction in man after aspirin ingestion. *Lancet* **ii**: 495–7.

Weiss H J. (2003) Historical sketch: the discovery of the antiplatelet effect of aspirin: a personal reminiscence. *Journal of Thrombosis and Haemostasis* **1**: 1869–75.

White H D, Norris R M, Brown M A, Brandt P W, Whitlock R M, Wild C J. (1987a) Left ventricular end-systolic volume as the major determinant of survival after recovery from myocardial infarction. *Circulation* **76**: 44–51.

White H D, Norris R M, Brown M A, Takayama M, Maslowski A, Bass N M, Ormiston J A, Whitlock T. (1987b) Effect of intravenous streptokinase on left ventricular function and early survival after acute myocardial infarction. *New England Journal of Medicine* **317**: 850–5.

Widdicombe J G. (1954) Respiratory reflexes excited by inflation of the lungs. *Journal of Physiology* **123**: 105–15.

Wilcox R G, von der Lippe G, Olsson C G, Jensen G, Skene A M, Hampton J R. (1988) Trial of tissue plasminogen activator for mortality reduction in acute myocardial infarction. Anglo-Scandinavian Study of Early Thrombolysis (ASSET). *Lancet* **ii**: 525–30.

Wilcox R G, von der Lippe G, Olsson C G, Jensen G, Skene A M, Hampton J R. (1990) Effects of alteplase in acute myocardial infarction: six-month results from the Anglo-Scandinavian Study of Early Thrombolysis (ASSET) study. *Lancet* **335**: 1175–8.

Wilcox R G, Hampton J R, Banks D C, Birkhead J S, Brooksby I A B, Burns-Cox C J, Hayes M J, Joy M D, Malcolm A D, Mather H G, Rowley J M. (1986) Trial of early nifedipine in acute myocardial infarction: the Trent study. *British Medical Journal* **293**: 1204–8.

Willis A L, Smith J B. (1981) Some perspectives on platelets and prostaglandins. *Progress in Lipid Research* **20**: 387–406.

Weismann R E, Tobin R W. (1958) Arterial embolism occurring during systemic heparin therapy. *American Medical Association: Archives of Surgery* **76**: 219–27.

Wright H P. (1941) Adhesiveness of blood platelets in normal subjects with varying concentration of anticoagulants. *Journal of Pathology and Bacteriology* **53**: 255–62.

Wright P. (2005) Obituary: Sir John Vivian Dacie. *Lancet* **365**: 1382.

Yusuf S, Peto R, Lewis J, Collins R, Sleight P. (1985a) Beta blockade during and after myocardial infarction: an overview of the randomized trials. *Progress in Cardiovascular Diseases* **27**: 335–71.

Yusuf S, Collins R, Peto R, Furberg C, Stampfer M J, Goldhaber S Z, Hennekens C H. (1985b) Intravenous and intracoronary fibrinolytic therapy in acute myocardial infarction: overview of results on mortality, reinfarction and side-effects from 33 randomized controlled trials. *European Heart Journal* **6**: 556–85.

Zallen D T, Christie D A, Tansey E M. (eds) (2004) The Rhesus Factor and Disease Prevention. *Wellcome Witnesses to Twentieth Century Medicine*, vol. 22. London: Wellcome Trust Centre for the History of Medicine at UCL. Freely available online under publications at www.ucl.ac.uk/histmed

Zapol W M, Qvist J. (eds) (1976) *Artificial Lungs for Acute Respiratory Failure: Theory and practice.* New York, NY; London: Academic Press; Washington, DC; London: Hemisphere.

Zawilska K M, Born G V R, Begent N A. (1982) Effect of ADP-utilizing enzymes on the arterial bleeding time in rats and rabbits. *British Journal of Haematology* **50**: 317–25.

Zimmermann N, Kienzle P, Weber A A, Winter J, Gams E, Schror K, Hohlfeld T. (2001) Aspirin resistance after coronary artery bypass grafting. *Journal of Thoracic and Cardiovascular Surgery* **121**: 982–4.

Zucker M B, Peterson J. (1968) Inhibition of adenosine diphosphate induced secondary aggregation and other platelet functions by acetylsalicylic acid ingestion. *Proceedings of the Society for Experimental Biology and Medicine* **127**: 547–51.

Zucker M B, Brownlea S, McPherson J. (1987) Insights into the mechanism of platelet retention in glass bead columns. *Annals of the New York Academy of Sciences* **516**: 398–406

Biographical notes*

Dr Y S (Mick) Bakhle
DPhil DSc (b. 1936) moved from the Oxford Department of Pharmacology, following John Vane and Gustav Born, to the department at the Royal College of Surgeons in 1965, leaving, as Reader, in 1993 to join the National Heart and Lung Institute, London. He is now Senior Research Fellow and Honorary Reader in Leukocyte Biology, Imperial College, London.

Professor Sune Bergström
(1916–2004) began research on lipid extracts of sheep vesicular suggested by Ulf von Euler in 1945. He joined the Karolinska Institute, Stockholm, as Assistant in the Biochemical Department in 1944. Following the war and a research fellowship at Basel University, he was appointed Professor of Physiological Chemistry at the University of Lund in 1947, returning in 1958 as Professor of Chemistry, to the Karolinska Institute, where he was Rector from 1969–77. He has been called the father of prostaglandins and is credited with the first breakthrough with his successful purification of two important prostaglandins and the identification of their chemical structure, showing they are produced from unsaturated fatty acids. He shared the 1982 Nobel Prize in Physiology or Medicine with his student Bengt Samuelsson and Sir John Vane. See http://nobelprize.org/medicine/laureates/1982/bergstrom-autobio.html (visited 18 October 2004).

Dr Hugh Blaschko
FRS (1900–93), biochemist, qualified at the University of Freiburg in Breisgau, Germany, and worked at University College London from 1929–30 and 1933–34 and at the Physiological Laboratory, Cambridge University, from 1934 to 1944 where he joined Professor Joseph Barcroft at the Department of Physiology and gained his PhD. He was invited to Oxford by Professor J H Burn in 1944. He eventually became Reader in Biochemical Pharmacology, Oxford University, later Emeritus and was Emeritus Fellow of Linacre College, Oxford, from 1967 until his death. See Blaschko (1983).

*Contributors are asked to supply details; other entries are compiled from conventional biographical sources.

Professor Sir Christopher Booth Kt FRCP (b. 1924) trained as a gastroenterologist and was Professor of Medicine at the Royal Postgraduate Medical School, Hammersmith Hospital, London, from 1966 to 1977 and Director of the Medical Research Council's Clinical Research Centre, Northwick Park Hospital, Harrow, from 1978 to 1988, and Harveian Librarian at the Royal College of Physicians from 1989 to 1997. He was the first Convenor of the Wellcome Trust's History of Twentieth Century Medicine Group from 1990 to 1996.

Professor Gustav Born FRCP HonFRCS FRS (b. 1921) was Vandervell Professor of Pharmacology at the Royal College of Surgeons from 1960 to 1973; Sheild Professor of Pharmacology at the University of Cambridge, Fellow of Gonville and Caius College, Cambridge, from 1973 to 1978 and Professor of Pharmacology at King's College London from 1978 to 1986, later Emeritus. He is currently at the William Harvey Research Institute, St Bartholomew's and the Royal London School of Medicine and Dentistry as Professor of Biochemical Pharmacology, at Queen Mary and Westfield College, London. He was the Founding President of the British Society of Haemostasis and Thrombosis from 1979 to 1981. The original aggregometer is in the Science Museum, London. He also has written about the life of his family in Born (2002b). See Figures 8, 14.

Professor Donald Chambers PhD (b. 1937) was trained at Columbia University, New York, and Harvard University, Cambridge, MA, and has held faculty positions at the University of California at San Francisco and the University of Michigan. He was Professor of Biochemistry and Molecular Genetics at the University of Illinois College of Medicine, Chicago, from 1985 to 2004, and head of the department. His research interests have evolved from platelet biology to neuro-immune interactions with particular emphasis on molecular medicine. He was Visiting Scholar, Green College, Oxford, from 1989 to 1993 and Honorary Visiting Fellow since 1993. Since 2000 he has been a Senior Research Associate at the Wellcome Unit for the History of Medicine, Oxford.

Professor Archie Cochrane CBE MBE FRCP FFCM (1909–88), medical scientist and epidemiologist, whose first clinical trial was conducted as a prisoner of war in Salonika. Following the war he was appointed to the Medical Research Council's Pneumoconiosis Research Unit in 1948. In 1960 he was appointed David Davies

Professor of Tuberculosis and Diseases of the Chest at the Welsh National School of Medicine, Cardiff, becoming Director of the Epidemiology Research Unit there in 1961 until his retirement in 1974. His papers are available for study at the Cochrane Archive, Llandough Hospital, Penarth, Cardiff. See Cochrane (1976); Cochrane [ALC] (1988).

Professor Sir John Dacie
Kt FRCP FRS (1912–2005), an influential haematologist who established the study of the blood and its diseases as a laboratory and a clinical speciality. Following war service in the Royal Army Medical Corps, he was appointed Senior Lecturer in Clinical Pathology, later Reader in Haematology at the Royal Postgraduate Medical School, Hammersmith Hospital, London, from 1946 to 1956, and Professor of Haematology there from 1957 until his retirement in 1977, later Emeritus. See Anon. (2005); Wright (2005). See also the 1991 interview with Sir John Dacie by Sir Christopher Booth [videorecording]. Oxford: Oxford Brookes University, held as 1795v, Medical Film & Audio Library, Wellcome Library, London.

Dr Hewan Dewar
MD FRCP (b. 1913) was Honorary Consultant, Physiology and Cardiology, at the Royal Victoria Infirmary, Newcastle, from 1947 to 1978. See Dewar (1998).

Professor John Dickinson
FRCP (b. 1927) was trained at Oxford and University College Hospital (UCH), London, and appointed Physician at UCH in 1964, then Professor of Medicine at St Bartholomew's Hospital Medical College, London, from 1974 to 1992. He is now Emeritus Visiting Professor at the Wolfson Institute of Preventive Medicine, London. He has been a member of the MRC, Chairman of the British Medical Research Society, and Secretary of the European Society for Clinical Investigation. He retains a strong interest in clinical research and in the aetiology of disease.

Professor Sir Richard Doll
Kt CH OBE FRCP FRS (b. 1912) qualified in 1937 from St Thomas' Hospital Medical School, London. After serving in the war, he joined Sir Francis Avery Jones in 1946, working on peptic ulcer, and in 1948 joined Sir Austin Bradford Hill's MRC Statistical Research Unit, which he directed from 1961 to 1969 and was subsequently Regius Professor of Medicine at the University of Oxford from 1969 to 1979, later Emeritus. He was Chairman of the Adverse Reaction Subcommittee, Committee on Safety of Medicines,

from 1970 to 1977 and has been Honorary Consultant, Imperial Cancer Research Fund Cancer Studies Unit, Radcliffe Infirmary, Oxford, since 1983.

Professor Peter Elwood FRCP (b. 1930) was a member of the scientific staff of the Epidemiological Research Unit (South Wales) from 1963, succeeding Archie Cochrane as its Director in 1974 until his retirement in 1995. He qualified in medicine in Queen's University Belfast in 1954, where he worked with John Pemberton from 1958 to 1963. He holds an Honorary Professorship in the Department of Epidemiology, Statistics and Public Health Medicine in the University of Wales College of Medicine and the Department of Social Medicine in the University of Bristol and is a Visiting Professor in the Department of Science in the University of Ulster. See Ness *et al.* (2002).

Professor Ulf von Euler (1905–83) was Professor of Physiology at the Karolinska Institute in Stockholm, Sweden, from 1939 until 1971. He had been awarded a Rockefeller Fellowship and spent some time with Henry Dale during 1930–31. Following the discovery of Substance P, von Euler subsequently discovered prostaglandin and vesiglandin (1935), piperidine (1942) and noradrenaline (1946). He shared the 1970 Nobel Prize in Physiology or Medicine with Sir Bernard Katz and Julius Axelrod 'for their discoveries concerning the humoral transmitters in the nerve terminals and the mechanism for their storage, release and inactivation'. See Blaschko (1985); http://nobelprize.org/medicine/laureates/1970/index.html (visited 9 September 2004).

Professor Rod Flower FMedSci FRS (b. 1945) became a member of staff at the Wellcome Foundation in 1973, and was senior scientist with the Department of Prostaglandin Research at the Wellcome Research Labs, Beckenham, Kent, from 1975 to 1984. He was Professor of Biochemical Pharmacology at the University of Bath from 1984 and head of the School of Pharmacy and Pharmacology from 1987, until he moved to St Bartholomew's and The Royal London School of Medicine and Dentistry as Professor of Biochemical Pharmacology at Queen Mary and Westfield College, London, in 1989 where he was head of the Division of Pharmacology from 1998 to 2003, and has been a Director and founding member of the William

Harvey Research Institute there since 1989. He has been associated with both Sir John Vane and Gus Born for much of his professional life, and has a major interest in the aspirin-like drugs, inflammation, platelets and thrombosis.

Professor Alison Goodall
PhD (b. 1949) worked at the Royal Free Hospital School of Medicine, London, from 1972 to 1997, moving to the University of Leicester in 1997 as non-clinical Lecturer, then Reader in the Department of Pathology. She has been Professor of Thrombosis and Haemostasis in the Department of Cardiovascular Sciences at the University of Leicester since 2003.

Professor John Hampton
FRCP FESC FFPM (b. 1937) trained at Oxford and worked with Professor J R A (Tony) Mitchell in Professor Pickering's department from 1964 to 1968. He was Professor of Cardiovascular Medicine, later Emeritus, at Queen's Medical Centre, Nottingham, from 1974 until his retirement in 1998.

Professor Roger Hardisty
FRCP (1922–97) trained in clinical pathology at St Thomas' Hospital, London, concentrating on haematology, particularly the bleeding disorders. He was Consultant Haematologist to the Hospital for Sick Children, Great Ormond Street, London, from 1958 to 1988 and Professor of Paediatric Haematology at the Institute of Child Health, University of London, from 1969 to 1987. He established the first paediatric haematology department in the UK at Great Ormond Street, and also ran a major centre for the treatment of haemophilia and similar disorders. His own interests were in platelets and latterly in the childhood leukaemias. See Weatherall and Lock (1997). See also Christie and Tansey (2003), 30–1, 46.

Professor Michael Harrison
DM FRCP (b. 1936) trained in London and Oxford, where he worked on inhibitors of platelet aggregation. In 1973 he became Consultant Neurologist at the Middlesex Hospital, London, and later at the National Hospital, Queen Square, London. He was awarded a personal chair at the Royal Free and University College Medical School, London, in 1988. His research interests are in stroke, the cerebral complications of cardiac surgery and the neurology of HIV infections and AIDS.

Professor Stan Heptinstall
PhD MBE (b. 1946) trained in chemistry before moving to Nottingham in 1972 to work on

platelets as a postdoctoral research fellow, later Lecturer (1975–85), Senior Lecturer (1985–90), Reader (1990–94) and has been Professor of Thrombosis and Haemostasis there since 1994. He was appointed editor-in-chief of the new journal, *Platelets*, in 1990 and has continued in that role to the present day.

Dr Arthur Hollman
MD FRCP (b. 1923) was a cardiologist at Hammersmith Hospital, London, when the first open-heart operations were done in 1957. Subsequently he was on the staff of Great Ormond Street Hospital for Children, London, and University College Hospital, London. Dr Hollman is the official archivist of the British Cardiac Society.

Dr Peter Hunter
MRCP (b. 1938) qualified from Middlesex Hospital, London, in 1963 and was Consultant Physician at the Royal Shrewsbury Hospital, from 1974 to 1993. From 1994 to 1997 he read pharmacology at King's College London as preparation for full-time research on the history of discovery of drugs and medicines in the modern era.

Professor Desmond Julian
CBE (b. 1926) trained in cardiology. He was Professor of Cardiology at the University of Newcastle upon Tyne from 1975 until his retirement in 1986, later Emeritus. From 1986 until 1993 he was the Medical Director of the British Heart Foundation. His research was mainly in the field of coronary heart disease and he was the first to propose the concept of the coronary care unit. He was President of the British Cardiac Society from 1985–87 and Vice-President of the Royal College of Physicians from 1991–92.

Dr Peter MacCallum
FRCP FRCPath (b. 1958) trained in haematology in Manchester and London, Since his appointment to St Bartholomew's and the Royal London. Since his appointment in 1995 he has been a Senior Lecturer in Haematology at St Bartholomew's Hospital (Bart's) and The London, Queen Mary's School of Medicine and Dentistry, London, and Honorary Consultant Haematologist at Bart's and The London NHS Trust, London.

Dr Martyn Mahaut-Smith
PhD (b. 1962) Following postdoctoral studies (1987–92) in Bristol, Cambridge, Toronto and San Diego, CA, he returned to Cambridge, held a British Heart Foundation Science Lectureship at the University of Cambridge from 1992 and has been a Senior Lecturer in Physiology since 2004.

Professor Thomas Meade
CBE FRCP FMedSci FRS (b. 1936) was Director of the MRC Epidemiology and Medical Care Unit from 1970, first at Northwick Park Hospital, Harrow, later at the Wolfson Institute of Preventive Medicine when it moved in 1992. He retired from the MRC in 2001 and is Emeritus Professor of Epidemiology at the London School of Hygiene and Tropical Medicine.

Professor Denis Melrose
MRCP FRCS (b. 1921) was Professor of Surgical Science at the Postgraduate Medical School, London, and Surgical Registrar at the Hammersmith Hospital, London, from 1968 to 1983, later Emeritus. See Melrose (1953); Melrose *et al.* (1953); Cleland *et al.* (1968).

Professor J R A (Tony) Mitchell
(1928–91) was Foundation Professor of Medicine at the University of Nottingham, from 1968 to 1990. See H(ampton)JR (1991); Mitchell (1987). See also Figure 9.

Professor Salvador Moncada
FRCP FMedSci FRS (b. 1944) trained as a medical doctor in El Salvador, then did a PhD at the Royal College of Surgeons, London. From 1975 to 1996 he was at the Wellcome Research Laboratories, Beckenham, Kent, where he was Director of Research from 1985. He moved to University College London where he has been Director of the Wolfson Institute for Biomedical Research since 1996. See Figure 12.

Dr Robin Norris
MD FRCP FRACP FAHA (b. 1931) trained at the Universities of Otago, New Zealand, and Birmingham, and was Cardiologist in charge of the coronary care unit at Green Lane Hospital, Auckland, NZ, from 1967 until his retirement in 1992, and tenured investigator for the New Zealand Medical Research Council from 1970 to 1992. He has been Honorary Professor of Cardiovascular Therapeutics at the University of Auckland and Honorary Consultant Cardiologist at the Royal Sussex County Hospital, Brighton, and Director of the UK Heart Attack Study and a subsequent study based in Brighton from 1992–99, and Consultant to the UK Myocardial Infarction National Audit Project (MINAP) from 1999–2003. His interests are in acute coronary care, pathophysiology of MI and the epidemiology and clinical audit of ischaemic heart disease.

Dr John O'Brien
(1915–2002) haematologist, qualified in medicine at Oxford, later trained in haematology under Professor R G Macfarlane. O'Brien was among those who published the first description of Christmas Disease (now known as Factor IX deficiency, see Biggs *et al.* (1952)), and he went on to develop a method to measure how platelets form blood clots and contributed to the discovery that low-dose aspirin could reduce this. He was consultant haematologist at the South Devon and East Cornwall Hospital from 1945 to 1951 and at St Mary's Hospital, Portsmouth, until his retirement. See Elwood and Lewis (2002).

Professor Michael Oliver
CBE FRCP FRSE (b. 1925) was the Duke of Edinburgh Professor of Cardiology at the University of Edinburgh from 1976 to 1989, later Emeritus. He has been President of the British Cardiac Society from 1980 to 1984; of the Royal College of Physicians of Edinburgh from 1986 to 1988; and Director of the Wynn Institute for Metabolic Research from 1990 to 1994.

Professor Clive Page
PhD (b. 1958) trained as a pharmacologist and has been Director of the Sackler Institute of Pulmonary Pharmacology at King's College London, and Professor of Pharmacology at King's College London, since 1986.

Professor Sir William Paton
Kt CBE FRCP FRS (1917–93) was on the scientific staff of the National Institute for Medical Research from 1944 to 1952; Reader in Applied Pharmacology at University College Hospital, London, from 1952 to 1954; held the Vandervell Chair of Pharmacology, Royal College of Surgeons, London, from 1954 to 1959; and was Professor of Pharmacology at the University of Oxford and Fellow of Balliol College from 1959 until his retirement in 1983. He was a member of the MRC from 1963 to 1967 and a Trustee of the Wellcome Trust from 1978 to 1987. His papers are held in Archives and Manuscripts, Wellcome Library, London, as PP/WDP, with further papers in GC/68/ and GC/154/A/11.

Professor Sir Stanley Peart
Kt FRCP FMedSci FRS (b. 1922) was Professor of Medicine at St Mary's Hospital Medical School, University of London, from 1957 to 1987, later Emeritus. He has been Master of the Hunterian Institute, Royal College of Surgeons of England from 1988 to 1992; Trustee of the Wellcome Trust from

1975 to 1994, Deputy Chairman from 1991 until 1994 and Consultant from 1994 to 1998; and a Beit Trustee from 1986 to 2003. He delivered the Goulstonian Lecture in 1959, the Croonian Lecture in 1979, and was a Founder Member of the Academy of Medical Sciences in 1998.

Professor Brian Pentecost
OBE MD FRCP (b. 1934) qualified at St Mary's Medical School, London, in 1957, was Consultant Physician and Cardiologist at the United Birmingham Hospitals from 1965 until 1993, Dean of Postgraduate Medicine and Dental Education from 1987 to 1991 and Honorary Professor of Medicine from 1991 until his retirement in 1998, later Emeritus. He has been Advisor in Cardiology to the Department of Health's Chief Medical Officer, 1986–93, a member of the Committee on Safety of Medicines from 1984–89 and 1996–98, the Royal College of Physician's Linacre Fellow (Director of Training), 1991–94, and Medical Director of the British Heart Foundation, 1993–99.

Sir George Pickering
Kt FRCP FRS (1904–80) was an assistant for eight years in Sir Thomas Lewis's Department of Clinical Research at University College Hospital, London, moving to St Mary's Hospital Medical School, London, to head the Medical Unit in 1939. The MRC established a Group for Research on Body Temperature Regulation (later Unit) under his direction in 1954. He went to Oxford as Regius Professor of Medicine in 1956 until his retirement in 1969. He was a member of the University Grants Committee from 1944 to 1954, and of the MRC from 1954 to 1958. A collection of his papers, CMAC/PP/GWP, is held in Archives and Manuscripts, Wellcome Library, London. See Figure 10.

Professor Colin Prentice
MD FRCP (b. 1934) was a Lecturer in Medicine at the Glasgow Royal Infirmary between 1964 and 1971, with Professor Stuart Douglas and George McNicol. He was a research student in 1964–5 with Professor Oscar Ratnoff at Case-Western Reserve University, Cleveland, OH. In 1971 he became Senior Lecturer in Medicine in Glasgow and in 1983 he was appointed Professor of Medicine at Leeds General Infirmary and the University of Leeds, until his retirement in 2000, later Emeritus. He was a Wellcome Research Fellow between 1971 and 1975, funded by the Wellcome Trust.

Dr Armand James Quick (1894–1978), an American physician and physiologist, who developed three tests: a one-step test to measure the amount of prothrombin present in blood plasma to determine prothrombin clotting time; a liver function test; and an intravenous hippuric acid test for liver function. He drew attention to the effects of aspirin on haemostasis and was able to show that aspirin could prolong the skin bleeding time. [Quick (1966).]

Professor Tom Quinn MPhil RN FESC (b. 1961) has been Professor of Cardiac Nursing at Coventry University since 2003 and has been closely involved in the development of the National Service Framework for Coronary Heart Disease and the Myocardial Infarction National Audit Project. He is a past Chairman of the working group on cardiovascular nursing of the European Society of Cardiology.

Professor Peter Richardson FCGI FRS (b. 1935) has been Professor of Engineering and Physiology at Brown University, Providence, RI, since 1984.

Dr Stewart Sage PhD ScD (b. 1962) has been Reader in Cell Physiology at the Department of Physiology, University of Cambridge, since 2003, and Fellow and Tutor for Research Students and Director of Studies in Natural Sciences (Biological), at Queens' College, University of Cambridge, since 1987.

Professor Bengt Samuelsson (b. 1934) studied medicine and biochemistry at the Karolinska Institute. The structural work on prostaglandin was conducted there with Sune Bergström from 1959–62. He was appointed Professor of Medical Chemistry at the Royal Veterinary College in Stockholm in 1967, returning to the Karolinska Institute as Professor and Chairman of the Department of Physiological Chemistry from 1973 until his retirement. He shared the 1982 Nobel Prize in Physiology or Medicine with Sune Bergström and Sir John Vane. His interests have been in the transformation products of arachidonic acid, which led to the discovery of endoperoxides, thromboxanes and the leukotrienes, and his group has studied the chemistry, biochemistry and biology of these compounds and their role in biological control system. See http://nobelprize.org/medicine/laureates/1982/samuelsson-autobio.html (visited 18 October 2004).

Dr Belding Scribner
(1921–2003), nephrologist, developed the Scribner shunt in 1960 while working with Wayne Quinton and David Dillard. The shunt was made of Teflon, but never patented. He shared the Albert Lasker Award for Clinical Medial Research for 2002 with Willem Kolff, for the 'development of renal dialysis, which changed kidney failure from a fatal to a treatable disease, improving the lives of millions of patients'. See Couser (2003).

Dr Roger Smith
MB (b. 1945) has been Consultant Cardiologist at the University Hospital of North Tees since 1979, previously Senior Registrar at the Newcastle Teaching Hospitals from 1976 to 1979. He has been Secretary of the Royal College of Physicians of Edinburgh and their Vice-President.

Professor Andrew Stevens
FFPHM (b. 1954) has been Professor of Public Health at the University of Birmingham since 1997 and is also head of Department. His personal interests centre on health technology assessment and healthcare needs. He is Chairman of a NICE appraisals committee and co-director of the National Horizon Scanning Centre at the University of Birmingham. Before coming to Birmingham he was the first director of the National Coordinating Centre for Health Technology Assessment (NCCHTA) at the University of Southampton.

Dr Duncan Thomas
MD DPhil FRCPath (b. 1929) was Associate Professor of Medicine at Tufts University School of Medicine in Boston, MA, from 1963 to 1970. From 1976 until his retirement he was Head of the Department of Haematology at the National Institute for Biological Standards and Control (NIBSC), Potters Bar, Hertfordshire. See Bloom and Thomas (eds) (1987).

Professor Sir John Vane
Kt DPhil DSc FRS (1927–2004), pharmacologist, discovered the role of prostaglandins in the human body in response to illness and stress and later demonstrated aspirin's mechanism of action [Vane (1971)]. He shared the 1982 Nobel Prize for Physiology or Medicine with Sune Bergström and Bengt Samuelsson. A student in Professor J H Burn's laboratory at the University of Oxford, he gained his second BSc in Pharmacology in 1949, followed by a DPhil with Dr Geoffrey Dawes at the Nuffield Institute

for Medical Research, Oxford, and later held the Royal Society's Stothert Research Fellowship. He was Assistant Professor of Pharmacology at Yale University, Newhaven, CT, from 1953–55, moving to work with Professor Sir William Paton at the Royal College of Surgeons' Institute of Basic Medical Sciences, London, in 1955, first as Senior Lecturer, Reader and as Professor from 1966 to 1973. He became Group Research and Development Director at the Wellcome Foundation, Beckenham, Kent, from 1973 to 1985, moving to the William Harvey Research Institute as Director in 1986 and Chairman from 1990 until his death. He was also Professor of Pharmacology and of Medicine at the New York Medical College (1986–2004). See Anon. (2004). See also http://nobelprize.org/medicine/laureates/1982/vane-autobio.html (visited 18 October 2004) and a transcript of an interview with Max Blythe in Oxford, 24 February 1988 at www.brookes.ac.uk/schools/bms/medical/synopses/vane.html (visited 22 November 2004). Moncada (2005), also at www.nature.com/cgi-taf/DynaPage.taf?file=/nature/journal/v433/n7021/full/433028a_r.html&filetype=&dynoptions (visited 15 March 2005). See Figures 8 and 12.

Alfred Edward Webb-Johnson
Bt KCVO GCVO CBE FRCS (Baron Webb-Johnson of Stoke-on-Trent from 1948) (1880–1958), surgeon, was Hunterian Professor of Surgery and Pathology at the Royal College of Surgeons of England, 1917; Vice-President and Consulting Surgeon to the Middlesex Hospital, London, and Dean of the Middlesex Hospital Medical School from 1919 to 1925; Surgeon to HM Queen Mary from 1936 to 1953; President of the Royal College of Surgeons 1941 to 1948. See Anonymous (1958).

Dr John Yarnell
(b. 1945) worked as an epidemiologist at the Medical Research Council Epidemiology Unit (South Wales) from 1975 to 1993, initially in studies of respiratory disease and the health of women, but in 1979 initiated and worked extensively on the Caerphilly Collaborative Heart Disease Study. From 1993 he became Senior Lecturer in Cardiovascular Epidemiology at Queen's University Belfast, and a member of the MRC's Steering Committee on the Use of the Caerphilly Collaborative Database.

Glossary

Bold text within a definition indicates another glossary entry.

5-hydroxytryptamine (5-HT, also called serotonin)
A monoamine neurotransmitter also stored in non-neuronal tissue, including **platelets** where it is released during aggregation and is itself proaggregatory.

^{14}C-5-hydroxytryptamine (5-HT, also called serotonin)
A radio-labelled form of serotonin used to trace the distribution and metabolism of 5-HT (serotonin).

12-hydroxyheptadecatrienoic acid (HHT)
One of the three major metabolites of **arachidonic acid** in human **platelets** [12(S)-hydroxy-5Z,8E, 10E-heptadecatrienoic acid].

adenosine deaminase (ADA)
An enzyme involved in the production of inosine and ammonia. In the present context adenosine is an endogenous inhibitor of platelet aggregation and is produced by the breakdown of ADP released during platelet activation. Deamination of adenosine by ADA is one of the normal pathways of inactivating adenosine.

alteplase (*Actilyse*, Boehringer Ingelheim)
A streptokinase–plasminogen complex used to treat acute **MI**, and pulmonary embolism.

anistreplase (*Eminase*, Monmouth)
A **tissue plasminogen activator** produced by recombinant DNA technology used to treat acute **MI**.

antiphospholipid syndrome (APS)
A disorder characterized by recurrent arterial or venous thrombosis and associated with the presence of **lupus** anticoagulant or antiphospholipid antibodies.

arachidonic acid
An omega-6 fatty acid normally stored within the cell membrane and found only in animal fats. It is the precursor of **prostaglandins**, **prostacyclin** and **thromboxanes**. See Figure 15 on the next page.

aspirin (acetylsalicylic acid or ASA)
A non-steroidal anti-inflammatory analgesic that blocks the action of **cyclo-oxygenase** and prevents the production of **prostaglandins**, **prostacyclin** and **thromboxanes**. For platelets, the most relevant

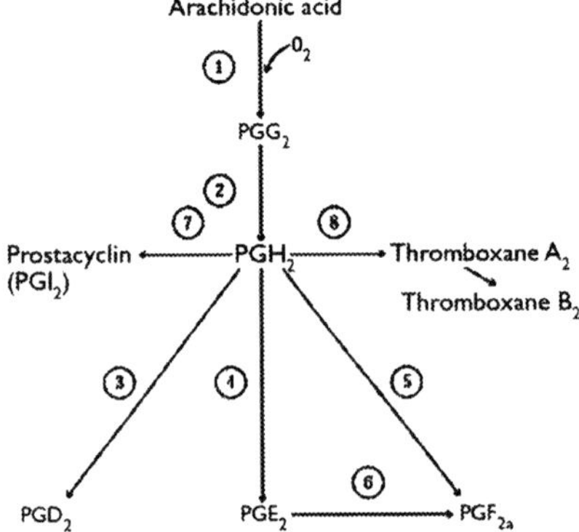

Figure 15: The metabolism of arachidonic acid to form prostaglandins, prostacyclin and thromboxanes.

Key to enzymes:

(1) prostaglandin synthase (cyclo-oxygenase)
(2) prostaglandin synthase (peroxidase)
(3) prostaglandin-H2 D-isomerase
(4) prostaglandin-H2 E-isomerase
(5) endoperoxide reductase
(6) prostaglandin-E2 9-reductase
(7) prostacyclin synthase
(8) thromboxane synthase

---

action is to prevent production of thromboxane A_2 by the **platelet** during aggregation, decreasing overall platelet aggregation. This is the basis of its use as prophylaxis against coronary thrombosis.

aspirin resistance

This usually refers to patients with coronary artery disease having ischaemic events despite receiving **aspirin**.

Bernard–Soulier syndrome

An autosomal recessive platelet disorder characterized by **thrombocytopaenia** with giant platelets.

β error, see type 2 error

bleeding-time (blood)

The blood issuing from a small puncture in the skin is called the bleeding time and bleeding normally stops in less than ten minutes.

blood oxygenators

Devices which take a flow of blood with a low oxygen content, usually venous blood, and by direct or indirect contact of the blood with a flow of oxygen-rich gas, discharge the blood with a higher oxygen content. They are used as artificial lungs, particularly during coronary artery bypass.

British Postgraduate Medical Federation (BPMF)
An association of postgraduate research Institutes located in London, mostly focused on a speciality: Orthopaedics (1946–87), Dental Surgery (1948–99, from 1992 as the Eastman Dental Institute), Psychiatry (1948–97), Child Health (1949–96), Neurology (1950–97), Urology (1951–88), and the **Institute of Basic Medical Sciences** (1941–86). It was disbanded in 1996, when the Institutes became constituent parts of the University of London. See www.lon.ac.uk/Colleges_Institutes/home.asp (visited 22 June 2005). See also the Institute of Basic Medical Sciences, Department of Pharmacology below.

C-reactive protein
A protein produced by liver cells in response to inflammation and used as a marker of an inflammatory state. See de Maat and Trion (2004).

cardiolipin antibodies
Their presence in human serum can be used in conjunction with other serological tests and clinical findings to assess the risk of thrombosis in individuals with **SLE** or lupus-like disorders. Anti-cardiolipin antibodies have been strongly associated with venous and arterial thrombosis.

Cardiothoracic Institute of the Brompton Hospital, London
See National Heart and Lung Institute, London.

Chédiak–Higashi syndrome
A rare and often fatal childhood autosomal recessive disorder, whose clinical characterization includes immune deficiency and decreased pigment in the eyes and skin compared to siblings. The patient bruises and bleeds easily as a result of deficient **platelets**.

clopidogrel (*Plavix*, Bristol-Myers Squibb, Sanofi-Synthelabo Ltd)
An analogue of ticlopidine that irreversibly modifies the **platelet** ADP receptor. It is an inhibitor of platelet aggregation and because it is not related to **aspirin** it can be used in patients with an intolerance, or with contra-indications, to **aspirin**.

cyclo-oxygenase (COX, also known as prostaglandin-endoperoxide synthase/synthetase (PGHS), fatty acid COX, and PGH synthase)
A key regulatory enzyme in the production of **prostaglandins**, **prostacyclin** and **thromboxane**. **Aspirin** [Vane (1971)] blocks the enzyme COX-1, first purified in 1976 and cloned in 1988. COX-2 [Vane *et al.* (1998); Smith *et al.* (2000a)] was identified in 1991,

and COX-3 in 2002 [Chandrasekharan *et al.* (2002)].

cyclic AMP (adenosine-3,-5 cyclic-monophosphate)
A second messenger that acts intracellularly to regulate various metabolic processes.

defibrillator
A machine producing an electric shock to stop cardiac fibrillation. During fibrillation the ventricular muscle does not contract adequately and cardiac output fails. The electric shock converts the fibrillation into normal contractions and cardiac output is restored.

dialysers
Also known as artificial kidneys, although not fully replacing kidney function, this machine brings the blood stream into contact with a flowing aqueous solution of salts through a hydrophilic membrane, resulting in progressive removal of dissolved substances in the blood up to molecular weights somewhat exceeding 1 kDa.

dipyridamole (*Persantin*, Boehringer Ingelheim)
A vasodilator launched in 1960 that decreases **platelet** adhesiveness thereby inhibiting the formation of clots in the arteries and used primarily in clinical practice as an antiplatelet agent. It interferes with platelet function by increasing the cellular concentration of **cyclic AMP** and increases coronary bloodflow.

disseminated intravascular coagulation (DIC)
An uncommon condition in which generalized intravascular blood coagulation occurs resulting in spontaneous bleeding.

ecto-AMPases, -ADPases, -ATPases
The AMP-, ADP-, and ATPases are enzymes (phosphatases) hydrolysing the terminal phosphate in each substrate.
Acting in sequence these enzymes can break down ATP to adenosine [see below] which can then be taken up into endothelial cells or be metabolized further by extracellular adenosine deaminase.

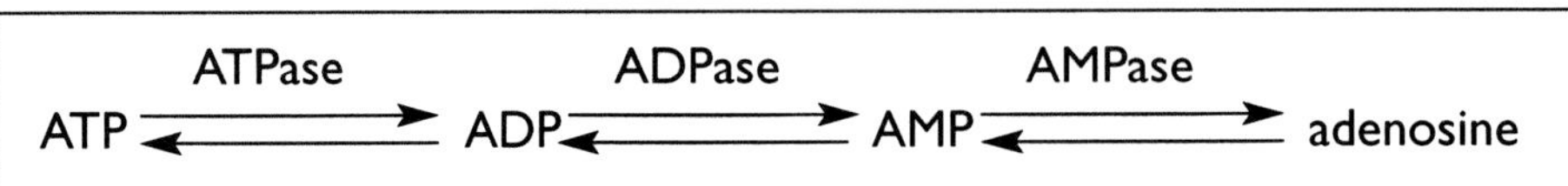

The prefix 'ecto' refers to the location of these enzymes on the outer surface of the cell membrane with free access to extracellular substrate. In the present context, ecto-ADPase on the luminal surface of the endothelial cell provides a mechanism for the rapid inactivation of proaggregatory ADP released from **platelets**.

ejection fraction

A measure of left ventricular function. The estimated volume of the left ventricle at end-diastole minus the volume at end-systole is expressed as a percentage of the end-diastolic volume. Normal ejection fraction is about 60 per cent; below 50 per cent is considered to indicate impairment.

electrophoresis

A technique used to separate a mixture of molecules by their differential migration through a gel in an electrical field. In platelets this provides a measure of the surface charge of platelets in diluted platelet-rich plasma.

factor VIII (antihaemophilic globulin)

A plasma coagulation factor whose inherited deficiency is responsible for the most common form of **haemophilia**.

fibrinogen

A circulating protein, which is the precursor of fibrin in clot formation.

fibrinolytic drugs

Drugs used to dissolve clots include **alteplase**, **anistreplase**, **reteplase**, and **streptokinase**.

firefly luminescence method

A method for estimating amounts of adenosine-triphosphate (ATP), by measuring the light generated by the reaction of the enzyme, firefly luciferase, with the ATP.

flow cytometry

The measurement of single cells as they flow, one cell at a time, through a beam of laser light. Their signals are picked up by detectors, converted for computer storage and data analysis to provide information about cell constituents and properties.

Glanzmann's thrombasthaenia

A genetic **platelet** disorder which leads to defective platelet aggregation and subsequent bleeding. The condition is rare and inherited in an autosomal recessive pattern.

glycoprotein (GPIIb/IIIa)
A conjugated protein, a component of the plasma membrane, that functions as a **platelet** receptor for fibrinogen and **von Willebrand factor** and plays an important role in platelet adhesion and aggregation.

haemophilia
A hereditary bleeding disorder which affects the clotting of blood. Patients with haemophilia A are deficient in **factor VIII** and those with haemophilia B are deficient in factor IX (Christmas disease).

haemostasis
The stopping of haemorrhage.

heparin
A glycosaminoglycan (mucopolysaccharide) anticoagulant found in mast cells, used *in vitro* to prevent blood clotting, and to treat venous and arterial thrombosis.

heparin-induced thrombocytopaenia (HIT)
An immune-mediated adverse drug reaction that may be associated with limb- or life-threatening thrombosis. The reaction occurs about five days into **heparin** treatment. The side-effects include deep vein thrombosis, pulmonary embolism, and disseminated intravascular coagulation. See Pentecost, page 111.

Hermansky–Pudlak syndrome (HPS)
An autosomal recessive genetic disorder described in 1959 that consists of visual and skin dysfunctions, prolonged bleeding time and defective platelet aggregation. Patients often have pulmonary fibrosis, granulomatous enteropathic disease which resembles Crohn's disease, and renal failure. HPS is frequent among Puerto Ricans. Further information can be found at http://falcon.roswellpark.org/HPSD/HPSD.htm (visited 31 January 2005).

HHT
See 12-hydroxyheptadecatrienoic acid

immune thrombocytopaenic purpura (ITP)
An immune disease that attacks **platelets**, reducing the platelet count (normal range is from 150 000 to 350 000 per millilitre) causing bleeding, bruises and tiny red dots (petechiae), on the skin.

indomethacin
An indole derivative with anti-inflammatory effects, more potent than **aspirin**, introduced in 1963 as an oral treatment for rheumatoid arthritis. Its use has been limited by its toxicity and its impairment of **platelet** function. It is also a robust inhibitor of the **cyclo-oxygenases**.

Institute of Basic Medical Sciences (IBMS), Department of Pharmacology
The department was established by the Royal College of Surgeons (RCS) in 1954 with Sir William Paton as Professor of Pharmacology. G V R Born was appointed the first Vandervell Professor of Pharmacology in 1959. From 1961 to 1984 the department was a constituent part of the IBMS, which had been a joint faculty of the RCS and the University of London since 1941 and was later part of the **British Postgraduate Medical Federation** (BPMF). The IBMS was disbanded in 1986 and most of the research departments closed, although some laboratories remained at Down House (Downe, Kent) under the RCS's newly created Hunterian Institute, discontinued by the RCS in 1993. Pharmacology, the last research department, closed in 1996. See also note 164.

International Society of Thrombosis and Haemostasis (ISTH)
Founded in 1954 in Basel, Switzerland, as the International Committee for the Standardization of the Nomenclature of the Blood Clotting Factors its name was later shortened to the International Committee on Thrombosis and Haemostasis (ICTH). The ISTH was organized in 1969 in the US and the ICTH acted as its working arm, renamed in 1987 as the Scientific and Standardization Committee (SSC) of the ISTH. A comprehensive nomenclature of quantities and units in thrombosis and haemostasis can be found at www.med.unc.edu/isth/ (visited 1 February 2005).

ischaemic heart disease (IHD, also coronary artery disease; coronary heart disease)
Heart dysfunction caused by narrowing of the coronary arteries.

lupus
see SLE

meta-analysis
A systematic review or overview that uses quantitative methods to summarize the results of many studies into one set of conclusions.

Michaelis–Menten kinetics
An equation that describes the relationship between the rate of an enzyme-catalyzed reaction and the concentration of free substrate.

myocardial infarction (MI, also heart attack)
The death of cardiac tissue following interruption of the blood, usually caused by obstruction of circulation due to thrombosis in a coronary artery. Infarction can result in permanent damage to an area of the heart.

National Heart and Lung Institute, London
Formerly the Cardiothoracic Institute of the Brompton Hospital, London, renamed as the Faculty of Medicine in 1991, affiliated to Imperial College London in 1996 and part of the Imperial College School of Medicine since 1997.

nitric oxide (NO)
Formerly known as endothelium derived relaxing factor (EDRF), NO is an important regulator of vascular and inflammatory functions; a key intermediate in the action of certain nitro-vasodilating compounds; and an inhibitor of platelet aggregation and an inducer of bronchodilatation.

paroxysmal nocturnal haemoglobinuria (PNH)
An acquired haemopoietic stem cell disorder which results in haemolytic anaemia or the increased destruction of red blood cells. A clinical characteristic is very dark urine (haemoglobinuria).

patch-clamp recording technique
An electrophysiological technique that allows the direct study of ion channel activity in membrane patches and small cells.

pentanoic acid
An aliphatic carboxylic acid containing five carbon atoms.

***Persantin*, see dipyridamole**

plasmin
An enzyme that digests fibrin, and thus dissolves blood clots.

plasminogen
A single-chain glycoprotein which is converted to **plasmin** when activated.

platelet
A blood cell that plays an important role in blood clotting. Once activated they can change shape, aggregate, and release several bioactive substances. Their properties of adhesion and aggregation facilitate haemostasis when the vascular endothelium is damaged, and also promotes clotting.

prostacyclin (PGI_2, also known as PGX)
A **prostaglandin** synthesized by endothelial cells lining the cardiovascular system. It is the most potent known inhibitor of **platelet** aggregation, a powerful vasodilator and opposes the actions of **thromboxane A_2**. It causes relaxation of arterial smooth muscle and inhibition of platelet aggregation, degranulation, and shape change, and is therefore thought to be important in maintaining vascular homeostasis.

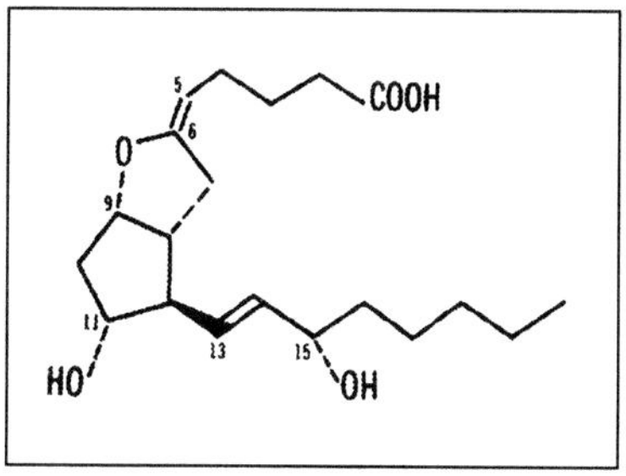

Figure 16: Structure of prostacyclin, 1978.

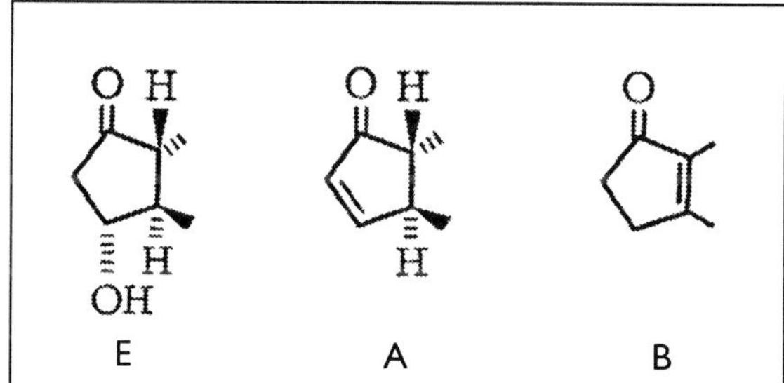

Figure 17: Structural differences between the E, A and B series prostaglandins.

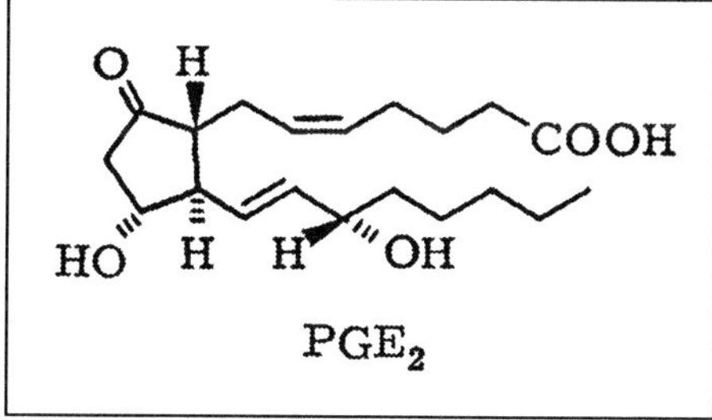

Figure 18: Structure of the prostaglandin PGE_2
(11α,15α-dihydroxy-9-oxo-5-cis-13-trans-prostadienoic acid)

prostaglandin (PG)

Any of a group of chemicals derived from unsaturated 20-carbon fatty acids, primarily **arachidonic acid** via the **cyclo-oxygenase** pathway. See Figures 17 and 18. See also COX.

Specific prostaglandins are designated by adding a letter to indicate the type of ring structure and a numerical subscript to indicate the number of double bonds in the hydrocarbon skeleton. For example, PGE_2 [Figure 18] causes vasodilation, inhibits gastic secretion, modulates inflammatory pain and oedema and induces fever. Most naturally occurring prostaglandins have two double bonds and their actions and effects vary with concentration, environment, and cell type.

rabbit aorta-contracting substance (RCS)
Now known as **thromboxane A_2** or TXA_2.

rare inherited platelet disorders,
See, for example, Bernard–Soulier syndrome; Glanzmann's thrombasthaenia; von Willebrand's disease.

reteplase
(*Rapilysin*, Boehringer Mannheim)
A recombinant **plasminogen** activator used to treat acute MI.

serotonin, see 5-hydroxytryptamine (5-HT)

streptokinase (*Kabinkinase*, Pharmacia & Upjohn; *Streptase*, Hoechst Marion Roussel)
An enzyme released by streptococci that converts **plasminogen** to plasmin, thus dissolving blood clots. Given intravenously it dissolves clots in venous thrombosis, pulmonary embolism and coronary thrombosis; it is also used with arteriovenous shunts and in acute **MI**. See Appendix 3.

systemic lupus erythematosus (SLE)
A long-lasting autoimmune disease that can affect virtually any system in the body. The immune system for unknown reasons becomes hyperactive and attacks normal tissue (may include the skin, joints, blood, lungs, kidneys, heart, brain and nervous system), causing inflammation, pain, and often organ damage.

thrombasthaenia
An autosomally inherited haemorrhagic disease with abnormalities of **platelet** function.

thrombin
An enzyme that induces clotting by the conversion of **fibrinogen** to fibrin.

thrombocytopaenia
A low **platelet** count often associated with haemorrhage.

thromboxane A_2 (TXA_2)
A lipid synthesized from arachidonic acid by COX with a chemical structure related to the **prostaglandins**, although having an endoperoxide ring instead of the five-carbon ring, an unstable, short-lived molecule.
Thromboxane A_2 is synthesized predominantly by **platelets** and induces vasoconstriction, platelet aggregation and bronchoconstriction in lung. Thromboxane A_2 degrades

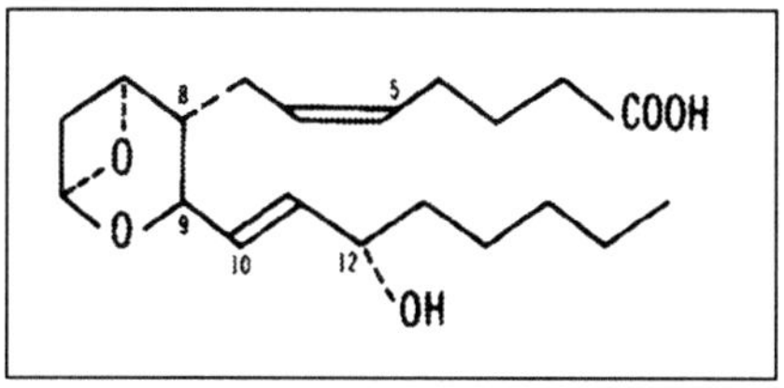

Figure 19: Structure of Thromboxane A_2, 1978.

spontaneously to the inactive TXB_2. See Figures 15 and 19.

tissue plasminogen activator (tPA; recombinant tissue plasminogen activator, rtPA)
An enzyme, serine protease, released from endothelial cells in response to signals including circulatory stasis produced by vascular occlusion. It binds to fibrin and converts **plasminogen** to plasmin. It is widely used in the treatment of acute MI, and if given within the first three hours of a thrombotic stroke, tPA may reduce permanent disability through the fibrinolytic action of plasmin.

type 2 error or β error in clinical trials
A statistical error, where the null hypothesis is accepted, giving a false negative result. The power of clinical trial is determined by the probability (β) of this error occurring, since this measures both the size of the trial and the amount of actual change in a particular subgroup.

von Willebrand's disease
An inherited bleeding disease resulting from a deficiency or abnormality of the von Willebrand factor, part of the plasma coagulation **factor VIII** complex. Clinical features include prolonged bleeding time and reduced **platelet** adhesiveness.

Index: Subject

Index: Names

Biographical notes appear in bold

Key to cover photographs

Front cover, top to bottom

Professor Tom Meade

Professor Gustav Born

Professor Rod Flower

Professor Salvador Moncada

Back cover, top to bottom

Professor Stan Heptinstall, Professor Peter Elwood
and Dr Duncan Thomas (row behind)

Professor Brian Pentecost

Professor John Hampton

Dr Hewan Dewar

CPSIA information can be obtained at www.ICGtesting.com
Printed in the USA
LVOW051612290512

283769LV00006B/150/A

9 780854 841035